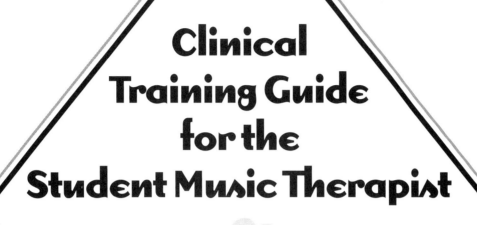

Clinical Training Guide for the Student Music Therapist

Second Edition

Donna W. Polen

Carol L. Shultis

Barbara L. Wheeler

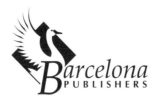

Barcelona PUBLISHERS

Clinical Training Guide for the Student Music Therapist:
Second Edition

Print ISBN: 9781945411168
E-ISBN: 9781945411175

Distributed throughout the world by:
Barcelona Publishers
10231 Plano Rd.
Dallas TX 75238

Website: www.barcelonapublishers.com
SAN 298-6299

Cover design: © 2016 Frank McShane

Permission

The authors thank the following for permission to reprint material in this book:

The American Music Therapy Association
    An adapted chart from Hadsell, N. A. (1993). Levels of external structure in music therapy. *Music Therapy Perspectives*, *11*(2), 61–65. doi:10.1093/mtp/11.2.61
    Portions of an assessment from Layman, D. L., Hussey, D. L., & Laing, S. J. (2002). Music therapy assessment for severely emotionally disturbed children: A pilot study. *Journal of Music Therapy, 39*(3), 164–187. doi:10.1093/jmt/39.3.164

Kenneth E. Bruscia
    General Behavior Checklist
    Strategy/Activity Form
    Guidelines for Activity Planning

Donna W. Polen
    Music Therapy Assessment for Adults with Developmental Disabilities

Carol L. Shultis
    Music Therapy Assessment and Initial Treatment Plan

Mary M. Wood
    A chart on stages of development in Developmental Therapy, from *Developmental Therapy* (1975), Baltimore, MD: University Park Press.

About the Authors

Donna W. Polen, LCAT, MT-BC, is Coordinator for Music Therapy at Finger Lakes Developmental Disabilities Service Office in Newark, NY, where she started the program in December 1980 and trained 79 interns. As adjunct Clinical Supervisor in the York Wellness and Rehabilitation Institute at Nazareth College in Rochester, NY, Donna supervises undergraduate and graduate music therapy students in their campus clinic placements. Donna also teaches clinical piano improvisation in the graduate program at the State University of New York at Fredonia and provides supervision for music therapy clinicians.

Donna's clinical practice has largely concentrated on work with adults with intellectual and developmental disabilities and related challenges such as autism, severe communication disorders, and dual diagnosis, including borderline personality disorder, bipolar disorder, and schizophrenia. She also has experience working with survivors of traumatic brain injury as well as with children and adults confronted with terminal illness, including amyotrophic lateral sclerosis and various dystrophies.

Donna presents extensively on her clinical work and occupational regulations. She co-authored a chapter in *Inside Music Therapy: Client Experiences* and contributed a chapter to *Guidelines for Music Therapy Practice in Developmental Health,* both from Barcelona Publishers.

Donna is active on state, regional, and national levels, serving the Mid-Atlantic Region (MAR) and AMTA in a variety of roles. As the MAR Representative to the Clinical Training Committee from 1987–2001, she co-authored the curriculum for the course for training directors and supervisors and served on the Professional Competencies Subcommittee of the Education Committee. She has served as an Assembly Delegate almost continuously since 1987. Donna has been serving as Chair of the New York State Task Force on Occupational Regulation since 2000, monitoring state licensure for creative arts therapists practicing psychotherapy, addressing issues of reimbursement, and overseeing the effort to achieve licensure for music therapists in the state. Donna has served AMTA in many roles, including as Council Coordinator and as a member of the Education and Training Advisory Board. Donna has received a number of awards, including the 2005 AMTA Service Award, the 2008 MAR Spirit of Unification Award, the 2012 AMTA Award of Merit, the 2012 AMTA Music Therapy Advocacy Founding Circle Award, and the 2014 MAR President's Award.

Carol L. Shultis, PhD, LPC, MT-BC, is Assistant Professor of Music Therapy, Converse College, Spartanburg, SC. She teaches and coordinates the clinical training for the undergraduate program. As a clinician in the Spartanburg Health System, she works primarily with pediatric and hospice patients. Converse students complete fieldwork in these settings under her supervision.

Carol served as Director of Music Therapy and Clinical Training Director for the Forbes Health System, Pittsburgh, Pennsylvania. She trained 88 interns and served as a clinical supervisor for over 100 Duquesne University music therapy students with additional music therapy students from Slippery Rock University and Seton Hill University. For 20 years, her work at the Forbes Health System included clinical services to psychiatric and medical/surgical patients in acute care; hospice families in inpatient and home care programs; and frail elderly, chronically ill, and rehabilitation patients in long-term care. She maintained a small private practice in the Bonny Method of Guided Imagery and Music after completing training in 1994. While working on her PhD and teaching at Seton Hill University, she offered music therapy to children and adolescents in partial hospitalization and at-risk middle school students and continued to work in long-term care.

Carol presents at many conferences and offers continuing education programs for music therapists, is published in *Psychiatric Times,* and co-authored Medical Music Therapy for Adults in *Music Therapy Handbook* (2015).

Carol served the music therapy profession as Advisor to the Mid-Atlantic Chapter of the National Association for Music Therapy (NAMT) student group (1983–1995), as Advisor to the Executive Board of the NAMT student organization from 1985–1996, and as member (1983–1985) and Chair (1985–1996) of the NAMT Student Affairs Advisory Board. She was Historian for the Mid-Atlantic Chapter from 2006–2013, a member of the AMTA Ethics Board 2006 - 2018, serving as co-chair since 2015 and currently serves on the Continuing Education Committee of the Southeastern Regional Chapter and as Coordinator of Continuing Education for the Music Therapy Association of South Carolina. Carol received the Service Award from the Mid-Atlantic Region of the AMTA in 2012.

Barbara L. Wheeler, PhD, MT-BC, retired in 2011 from the University of Louisville, Kentucky. She was previously on the faculty of Montclair State University, New Jersey, whence she received the designation of Professor Emerita.

Barbara has been active in music therapy since 1969, and her clinical work has been with children and adults with a variety of problems. She worked in three state hospitals with adults with emotional disorders and addictions and was employed at two different schools for children with special needs. She worked at the Creative Arts Rehabilitation Center in New York City, directed by Florence Tyson; studied at the Nordoff-Robbins Music Therapy Center at New York University with Clive and Carol Robbins; became a Certified Paraverbal Therapist under Evelyn Heimlich; and studied Neurologic Music Therapy (NMT) and became an NMT Fellow (Emeritus). In addition to being a music therapist, she is a licensed psychologist in New York.

Barbara has written a number of articles and chapters on music therapy, and her research interests and publications include both quantitative and qualitative research. She edited *Music Therapy Handbook, Music Therapy Research: Quantitative and Qualitative Perspectives, Music Therapy Research* (2nd edition), and *Music Therapy Research* (3rd edition, with K. Murphy).

Barbara is Past President of the American Music Therapy Association (AMTA) and was previously Chair of the Council on Education and Training of the World Federation of Music Therapy. She is on editorial and advisory boards of several journals and was both a discussion co-editor and interview co-editor for *Voices: A World Forum for Music Therapy.* She was honored with the 1999 Publication and Research Award given by AMTA, the 2005 Service Award given by the Southeastern Region of AMTA, the President's Award in 2013 from the Mid-Atlantic Region of AMTA, and an Award of Merit in 2016 from AMTA. She frequently speaks and consults about music therapy around the world. She has current faculty appointments at the University of Applied Sciences Würzburg Schweinfurt, Department of Social Studies, Würzburg, Germany, and the Karol Szymanowski Academy of Music, Katowice, Poland.

Table of Contents

Introduction:
How to Use This Book

We are pleased that you are reading this book, *Clinical Training Guide for the Student Music Therapist,* 2nd edition. We hope and expect that it will make your journey toward becoming a music therapist stimulating and rewarding.

This book is designed for use by music therapy students at all levels of training. We recognize that clinical training progresses as students move through their education and clinical experiences, and that students have different needs at each level. On the other hand, many of the same issues must be dealt with at each level. To attempt to meet these needs, we have organized the information in such a way as to encourage the scaffolding of knowledge and skills as you advance through typical levels of involvement: observing the music therapy session; participating and assisting as a student therapist; planning, co-leading, and—finally—leading the session. We expect students will use the book in different ways at each level, adapting it to their unique experiences and needs. We have structured the chapters to facilitate this, including suggestions for assignments, journaling, and discussion at the end of each chapter. The levels of involvement reflect the gradually increasing involvement and levels of responsibility of students as they progress through their music therapy training, from the first clinical observations through the internship. It is up to individual instructors and students to determine how quickly students move through these levels, both in terms of the use of the materials and resources in this book as well as in clinical placements. Considerations include the structure of the university program, the student's strengths and confidence, whether or not a music therapist is available as an on-site supervisor, and whether and how much a faculty member is available to supervise.

Because many of the issues that a student or therapist deals with are the same at each level of involvement, we encourage students to go through the book and suggested assignments several times, focusing differently based on current coursework and clinical placements. Students may find it helpful to use some chapters such as Client Assessment, Goals and Objectives, and Planning and Implementing Music Therapy Strategies as resources when working on session plan design for both class assignments and clinical site sessions. Faculty will, of course, decide exactly how to utilize this book and each chapter. We suggest, though, that chapters be read and discussed several times as the student moves through the clinical training process, with different emphases at each point.

This book is designed to meet the needs of music therapy students in the United States, although it may be used by students in other countries provided that philosophies of training are similar. Graduates of music therapy programs in the U.S. are expected to meet the AMTA *Professional Competencies* (American Music Therapy Association, 2013a). Material throughout the book will help students to meet the competencies.

Because music therapy students must be ready to work with any population, this book is applicable to a diverse array of clientele. In some parts of the book, examples are provided for specific clientele. In others, the student, clinical supervisor, and instructor will make the specific connections. Some terms and conventions are different from setting to setting. Knowing that this is the case, we have tried to address these differences in some areas, but in others the adaptations will have to be made by the reader. In general, we have used *client* and *clients* to refer to the people with whom music therapists work; exceptions to this are when those receiving services are referred to in a different way in a particular setting (for example, *patients* in a medical setting).

We hope this book will be your companion on your exciting journey toward becoming a music therapist, and that it will help you to acquire the skills that you need to make this journey as productive and positive as possible.

Clinical Training Guide for the Student Music Therapist

Second Edition

Doing Music Therapy: An Exploration

You are on your way to becoming an effective music therapy clinician—what an exciting path! The potential for music to help uplift and heal has motivated you to commit to your training and is why you are reading this book.

Becoming a music therapist takes time. Becoming a therapist is a process. As you learn and grow throughout your educational career and early years of work in the field, you will enjoy many peak moments and a measure of frustration as well. Don't worry, though: It's all part of learning what music therapy *is*, what it means to *do* it, and what it means to *be* a music therapist.

Before beginning any clinical work as a student therapist, it is helpful to understand the fuller context of your work, which involves consideration of (a) what it means to do any kind of therapy, (b) what it means to do music therapy, and (c) what is involved in the therapy process. This chapter is organized around these three considerations.

A first step in understanding what it means to do therapy involves developing a concept of health and wellness. With a clear understanding of this (grounded in knowledge of yourself), you are ready to consider the second step: how a therapist can help to optimize health and wellness. The third step is to develop a working definition of music therapy and understand some of the theories behind it. The therapy process involves knowledge of the potentials and challenges associated with a condition or diagnosis; assessment skills; treatment planning skills; implementation skills, including clinical musicianship; documentation skills; and interpersonal skills to work with clients and their significant others, staff, and community. It also includes our ethical thinking, our ability to self-monitor, and our willingness to continue to grow personally and musically.

All of this information is helpful in learning what music therapy is and how to do it. Doing music therapy also requires the development of an understanding of the therapeutic use of the self. Taylor (2008) described six modes of interaction with clients used by therapists rated as excellent clinicians by peers. These include advocating, collaborating, empathizing, encouraging, instructing, and problem solving. No one is naturally good at all of these, but therapists can develop skill in these modes. Clients will respond to different modes based on their unique personality traits, so each mode a therapist learns to use will help him or her relate to more clients.

Doing therapy, with or without music, is a complex process. Many factors affect the way in which music therapy is provided. How a treatment team understands what music therapy can offer to a given client may affect what you, the music therapist, are able to achieve with that client. Part of your job will be to educate the team about what is happening in your sessions, how it is benefiting your clients, and how music therapy might help other clients. Being a music therapist also means being an advocate for your clients and your profession.

As therapists, we bring to our work preconceived notions (which may or may not be accurate) about the importance of therapy. All therapists have ideas about engaging the client in therapy and how that might be accomplished. We all have ideas about the role the therapist plays in the process and the roles of family, friends, physicians, administrators, and staff from other disciplines. Music therapists also have notions about the role of music in music therapy. As professionals, music therapists have a responsibility to continually examine our work and approaches and to continue the process of self-growth—which, for a music therapist, includes musical growth.

If you are just embarking on your journey to becoming a music therapist, you may not yet grasp all of these ideas. In a first clinical experience, it is important to begin to understand what it means to interact with clients, to notice your personal responses to clients and therapy processes, and to observe how staff and family members perceive music therapy. In your initial clinical experience, you may be observing only—take advantage of this opportunity to really pay attention to what the therapist is doing, including their use of music and how the clients are responding. Read about the population or diagnostic group to develop an understanding of what it means to be a child with a developmental disability, an adult with a physical disability, or an older person experiencing loss. But, first and foremost, begin to become aware of what therapy is, how it is done, why it is done, who a therapist is, and what kind of a therapist you hope to become.

Understanding Therapy

Let us begin our discussion of what therapy is by realizing that all therapy is about change and growth. It is about assisting a client to function more fully within his or her potentials. It is a process facilitated by a therapist that, when effective, results in positive outcomes for the health and well-being of the client.

From a more psychological perspective, therapy can be described as a process that helps clients to (a) explore self and situations, (b) come to a deeper understanding of each, and (c) move to action (Egan, 1975). Dobson (1988) further describes therapy as:

> Teaching people, notably in groups, how to lead effective lives by mastering the continuing challenges of development. When that development is disrupted by particular concerns, "therapists" help alleviate those problems … they not only make certain that clients acquire the knowledge and skills to prevent or overcome similar problems in the future, but also help clients increase their general psychological effectiveness. (p. 210)

Ivey and Simek-Downing (1980) suggest that, in order to respond flexibly and creatively to another human being, we need to develop our understanding of several psychological theories and more than one worldview. Bruscia (2011), in the Sears Distinguished Lecture at the American Music Therapy Association annual conference, clearly defined the need for music therapists to understand our work from different perspectives and to develop the ability to shift from one view to another to meet client needs. Ultimately, he suggests we learn to think in a more integral way, thinking in the way that each client needs us to think. This suggests that, in your development as a music therapist, you will be well served by reading, considering, and embracing as many new perspectives as you can, allowing your worldview to continually develop and become more flexible.

In addition, as you develop as a music therapist, consider the value of undergoing your own personal therapy. In a discussion of growth theory, Maslow (1999) states, "only the one who respects health can do therapy" (p. 61). He refers to the concept of *active experiencing*, which is characterized by physical, emotional, and intellectual self-involvement; a recognition and ongoing exploration of one's abilities; the finding of one's own pace and the acceptance of that pace in not taking on too much at once; gains and improvements in skills that can be transferred to various tasks; and the opportunity that arises as a result of active participation to discover and uncover new interests and potentials.

As therapists, of course we want our clients to experience these things, but they also hold value for *you* in your own development as a therapist. The AMTA *Professional Competencies* (American Music Therapy Association, 2013a) speak directly to the importance of such ideas. These competencies include the ability to:

- Recognize the impact of one's own feelings, attitudes, and actions on the client and the therapy process;
- Establish and maintain interpersonal relationships with clients and team members that are conducive to therapy;
- Use oneself effectively in the therapist role in both individual and group therapy, for example, with appropriate self-disclosure, authenticity, empathy, and so forth, toward affecting desired behavioral outcomes;
- Accept criticism/feedback with willingness and follow through in a productive manner;
- Resolve conflicts in a positive and constructive manner;
- Express thoughts and personal feelings in a consistently constructive manner;
- Demonstrate critical self-awareness of strengths and weaknesses;
- Participate in and benefit from multiple forms of supervision (peer, clinical).

Understand that knowing yourself and your abilities and potentials and being willing to continue growing are crucial to your development as a therapist.

Understanding Music Therapy

We begin this section by first looking at a definition of music therapy. We will then consider several theories that expand our understanding of music therapy and how and why it works.

Definition

Perhaps Bruscia's (2014b) definition will help you to examine your own ideas about the field. It can also help you to begin to appreciate the benefits and limits of a working definition so that you can change it to reflect your ongoing experience and learning. Music therapy is, according to Bruscia, "a reflexive process wherein the therapist helps the client to optimize the client's health, using various facets of music experience and the relationships formed through them as the impetus for change. As defined here, music therapy is the professional practice component of the discipline, which informs and is informed by theory and research" (p. 36). This definition takes into account the following:

- Music therapy is reflexive—it is not a static event but requires ongoing evaluation and modification on the part of the therapist;
- It is a process—it takes place over time;
- The therapist helps the client—this clarifies the direction in which the help occurs;
- The goal is to optimize health—although *health* has various definitions, therapy is intended to make it better;
- Various facets of music experience are utilized—music therapy is centered on the use of music and specific music experiences, including listening, improvising, re-creating, and composing;
- Relationships are formed through these music experiences—these may be relationships between the client and the therapist and/or between the client and the music;

- The music and resulting relationships are the impetus for change—these changes may be personal (within the client), interpersonal (in relation to others), or ecological (in a sociocultural or physical environment);
- Music therapy is a discipline of professional practice—appropriately qualified therapists use music experiences and relationships to help clients, and our work is directly related to and impacted by our own unique body of theory and research.

This is a useful definition with which to begin and from which your growing understanding of music therapy can evolve. You may also find it very interesting to compare and contrast Bruscia's current definition with his original definition, "Music therapy is a systematic process of intervention wherein the therapist helps the client to achieve health, using musical experiences and the relationships that develop through them as dynamic forces of change" (1989, p. 47), and his second version, "Music therapy is a systematic process of intervention wherein the therapist helps the client to promote health, using music experiences and the relationships that develop through them as dynamic forces of change" (1998a, p. 20). As you will discover, the ongoing development of this definition is a tangible reflection of the changing worldview of Bruscia and subsequently a reflection of changes in the profession as a whole.

Theories

Some authors describe music therapy in terms of aesthetics, while others focus on meaning and still others view it from a scientific perspective. Aigen (1995) and Kenny (1989) speak of the importance of aesthetic considerations in music therapy work. Aesthetics and beauty play a major role in the outcome of the therapy process for these authors.

Aigen (1995) suggests that therapeutic progress is measured by changes in the aesthetic quality of the music and describes the importance of aesthetic expression as a focus for the client's emotional resistance that finds release in the rhythmic movement of the music (p. 250). He believes that this serves as a precursor for expressive and communicative development, and that it is this discharge of emotional resistance into expression that makes music therapy effective.

Kenny (1989) posits that, because the therapist and the client are aesthetic and the expression or communication of that aesthetic to the world is movement toward wholeness, music therapy is a pull toward wholeness created by the musical space between the therapist and the client. For Kenny, music provides a safe space for change, growth, and recovery. The therapist's role is to work with the client in the musical space in order to get to know one another, seeking the moment when a new field emerges, when the searching takes on a recurring form or "a particular tonality or dynamic, they *know* each other and there is security and confidence enough to initiate a sense of play and experimentation. At some point this experimentation bursts into an open space—*the field of play*" (p. 82). The therapist works musically with the client within this space, using experimentation, imitation, and modeling to encourage the client to reach beyond the safety of the familiar.

Other theoreticians look at the meaning that is inherent in music therapy. This meaning may be attributed to our participation in the creation of music. Creating music is deeply connected to our cultural heritage and our identity. In improvisational music-making, the dialogic nature of the experience is a source of meaning as well. For Ruud (1998), meaning is a result of the interaction between music-makers and their awareness of the influences of culture. Music therapy may lead to change in the self-concept of the client, allowing the client more possibilities for living in the world.

For Stige (2002), meaning in music therapy is co-constructed; in other words, it is based on both the client's and the therapist's *constructions* or understanding of what is occurring. Stige also sees meaning as culturally based and extends the practice of music therapy into the community as health promotion by embracing programs designed to lead to normalization of individuals typically excluded from community music-making. Stige describes music therapy as a culturally authorized form of ritual or repeated practice developed to help people with problems in living (p. 219). This ritual serves as a safe container for personal experiences and may be seen in relation to public and social functions.

Focusing on music therapy as a science and the need for music therapy to be research-based, Thaut (2000) describes a model for achieving therapeutic goals. The music therapy that Thaut finds valid is based upon scientific evidence and limits interventions to those that have been proven successful. This success is often found through research in related fields, with music experiences then being added in a parallel form. It is the music therapist's job to translate the nonmusical exercises that have been shown through research to achieve desired outcomes into parallel musical experiences, thus leading to music-based success in meeting stated goals (p. 12).

Bruscia (2011) posits that music therapy can be viewed through a scientific lens, as an art, or as a humanity. Each of these points of view addresses different components of the therapy process, and the choice of lens is a response to both the client's need and the therapist's understanding of the music therapy process. The therapist who is able to move between and among these modes in an integrative fashion is more able to address the client's immediate need for behavior change, the need to explore options for alternative responses, and the circumstantial needs to help the client make life choices or changes.

Stegemöller (2014) suggests that in order for music therapists to be successful in accessing financial and administrative support for services, we must become better skilled at explaining the ways in which neuroplasticity is impacted and activated through music therapy. Specifically, Stegemöller outlines a theoretical model of using brain neuroplasticity in music therapy to improve function in the areas of social interaction, emotional expression, cognitive development (learning or relearning skills), speech and communication, and movement (pp. 220–224).

The theories presented here are diverse and cover a range of ideas as to why music therapy works as it does. These and other theories help to provide a solid basis for understanding what music therapists do.

Choi (2008) conducted a survey of music therapists to inquire about their theoretical awareness of their practice. In reviewing literature, Choi identified a broad range of theoretical orientations adopted by music therapists, including behavioral, psychoanalytic, existential/humanistic, and music and medicine. The results of this survey revealed that, regardless of theoretical orientation, music therapists are dedicated to providing meaningful music experiences for their clients and often incorporate a variety of techniques and orientations in their work. The study also found that many music therapists base their work on their previous schooling. The importance of this for you, the reader, is to understand that schools cannot provide a complete and comprehensive background in all theoretical orientations, especially with the ever-growing range of ideas that are being explored. The responsibility lies with each of us to expand our knowledge base and to look at theories outside the field of music therapy as well as those indigenous to our discipline and our profession.

Understanding the Therapy Process

The basic structure of the therapy process involves identifying needs, planning interventions, and measuring outcomes. We usually speak of this as assessment, treatment planning, and evaluation. This process unfolds in incremental steps in some settings, although in short-term settings the steps may happen almost simultaneously. Following assessment, treatment planning involves the creation of goals and objectives, followed by the design of interventions or, in the case of music therapy, music experiences that will assist the client in moving toward the identified goals.

Finally, therapy is implemented and a process of evaluating targeted outcomes occurs. We will discuss and expand upon these processes throughout this book.

A number of books and other resources on the therapy process, written by authors outside of music therapy, are available (e.g., Benjamin, 2001; Corey, 2009; Frank & Frank, 1991). A different perspective is found in *How Can I Help? Stories and Reflections on Service* (Dass & Gorman, 1985) and is also recommended.

Knowing What to Do

In order to plan for a music therapy session for any client or group of clients, the music therapist must know the following: (a) client needs, (b) the therapist's role, and (c) how to use music. All of these topics are typically covered in music therapy coursework. If you are beginning your first practicum, you may not know much of this information yet and will need to ask questions and read and observe closely. If you are a more experienced student, you are in the process of developing a personal therapeutic style that will allow you to incorporate who you are with what you know into an approach to working with clients. If you are beginning your internship, you have most likely explored these areas in numerous formats and are now challenged to integrate that information into your therapeutic style as it continues to take form. If you are clear about what the client needs, how to help the client move toward the goals, and how to use music to facilitate that movement, you will know what to do during your sessions.

Identifying Client Needs

In order to work effectively with any client or group, the therapist must have a basic understanding of the needs of the client or group. Needs are both general (as indicated by the characteristics of a population or diagnostic group) and individual (as reflected by the unique life experiences of any given person). The normative characteristics of a client population will give the therapist a general sense of the questions to be formulated for the assessment process. Knowing the issues or problems that are common in a client population helps the therapist to define assessment experiences and to watch for specific kinds of responses and information, as well as providing hints for interacting with the client. For example, a therapist who understands the loss and the associated stress responses related to aging will hold that framework in mind when working with an aging person regardless of the person's diagnostic group. An older adult who has just had a cerebral vascular accident (stroke) and is receiving physical rehabilitation for the subsequent physical changes is also experiencing many losses and stressors. The therapist can more effectively understand how to intervene and contribute to the client's overall recovery if the effects of loss and stress are included in the planning process, in addition to the musical experiences that will help to develop fine motor control in the client's arm and hand.

Understanding a client's needs requires a thorough assessment of that person. During assessment, you will consider many factors, including strengths; needs or weaknesses; background information, including diagnosis or symptoms; current and previous treatment; musical experience and preferences; educational, social, and cultural background; mood; and any precautions that may affect music therapy interventions.

Understanding the Therapist's Role

Your role as a therapist in any given client's life is determined by a number of factors: the setting where the therapy is being provided, the other team members involved in treatment, and the level of intervention being offered (e.g., whether music therapy is serving as a primary therapy or as an adjunctive service). How you understand your role as a therapist and the personal qualities you bring to the therapeutic relationship also affect what you do.

In considering these factors, you might begin by looking at the setting in which music therapy is to be provided. While some generalizations can be made about the differences between outpatient versus inpatient or residential services, it is important to consider how each setting uniquely defines how services can be offered. For example, a once-a-week outpatient session with the music therapist may be a highlight of a client's week, but it represents a small fraction of the client's life, so the therapist will want to craft an intervention that can carry the client through to the next session. In spite of this fact, the music therapy session may be very important to the client. Music therapist Barbara Reuer, referring to a hospital music therapy session, speaks to how important a one-time visit can be:

> When you are doing bedside work at a hospital, most times it is a once-in-a-lifetime experience for the patient. How the therapist interacts with that patient is crucial. When you see patients and/or families in medical/hospice settings, every moment for them can be life-changing and forever memorable. Everything is augmented in their lives because of the intensity of what that person may be experiencing. One cannot underestimate the importance of a one-time visit. (personal communication, March 13, 2005)

The therapist may wish to provide at-home resources, exercises, or homework to extend the therapy process. In the case of children, adults with developmental delays, or others with disabilities, parents or caretakers can be taught skills to extend the benefits of music therapy interventions beyond the session. Whether music therapy is provided in a clinic or school setting or in the client's home (as is often the case in hospice work, for instance), the setting will impact the timing of treatment and the options available to the therapist. For example, the family of a hospice client being seen at home may be very protective of a client, limiting the time the therapist can spend in the home. This requires that the therapist choose a musical experience that fits the time frame available. Timing may also be affected as sessions are scheduled around a family's life, other therapies, and even the energy and endurance of the client.

When working in an inpatient setting, it is essential to consider the length of stay for the clients. When approaching a client for whom your first intervention is likely to be your only intervention, the student music therapist should use caution and respect. It is important to build rapport and trust but also to set limits on how much is done in a single session. What can you do—and what should you avoid doing so as not to leave the client hanging following a single encounter? This is quite different than building a relationship with a client over time, gently engaging the client with the music to move toward longer-range goals and allowing time for closure when your work together is drawing to an end.

When working at a residential facility, first find out how long clients live at the facility. Whether or not the clients are close to your age will also impact how you as a student music therapist relate to this population. You must also be careful to develop an understanding of the appropriate boundaries of a therapeutic relationship. A productive relationship with clients depends on clearly establishing therapeutic distance while at the same time building a bond of trust. Of course, this applies to all settings but becomes especially relevant in long-term situations.

All of these issues impact the *therapeutic use of self* in the music therapy process. Take time to consider how you relate to clients and how that relationship impacts the clients' responses to your music therapy interventions. This will help you to develop a therapeutic style that is unique to you while remaining within the boundaries of ethical and effective practice.

Another important aspect of being a music therapist is your relationship with the treatment team. Understanding how a given treatment team is structured is essential for understanding your role. Be sure to learn who else is working with the client and find out about the primary team goals for this client. It is also helpful to know who sets the goals: Is it a physician, a team leader, or the team in consultation with all members? It is also vital to know what role music therapy can play in helping the client to reach the goals within the context of this particular treatment team. In some settings, all team members work on team goals, while in others the team sets general goals and each therapist writes discipline-specific goals. What goals are you addressing as a student therapist, and how are these defined? You may be given specific goals to address by a supervisor, you may be asked to assess a specific client or group and set goals yourself, or you may use generic goals as you learn to select more specific goals as a part of your development as a music therapist.

In order to set appropriate therapeutic goals for any client or group, the therapist must understand not only the client's needs but also the implications of working toward a goal. How will this goal contribute to the overall quality of life for this client? Let us look at a common goal area that student therapists address: "socialization skills." How can changes in socialization make a difference for this person or persons? It might be that the ultimate value of increased social contact will be that the client is less isolated and withdrawn and less prone to symptoms of depression. Perhaps because of relationships built in a music therapy group, the client will be motivated to join in other programs and thus become more engaged in life. Another potential benefit for the client is the development of a more positive attitude toward the treatment process itself because of shared experiences with others undergoing similar treatment. By keeping these interrelated factors in mind, you will be able to set the most useful goals for the client. After considering these possible outcomes, the therapist may find that a more accurately stated goal is "interact with peers outside the group setting as observed on the unit." Another goal that may arise from thinking through these factors is "demonstrate increased motivation to participate in treatment." In this case, socialization skills are more clearly defined as the "sharing of thoughts or feelings about current treatment," which has led to a clearer and more measurable outcome.

The therapist must also consider the client's role in setting goals. Often, the client's role is affected by the therapeutic relationship. The therapist may also evoke goals from the client (or from the family or responsible party) that are more meaningful to the client than those the therapist would have created independently. It is important for the therapist to understand that interaction and relationship with the client or responsible party may affect this part of the goal-setting process as well as the delivery of services.

Finally, the therapist's understanding of the self and definition of therapy affects his or her work. The therapist's belief system can hinder rapport and effectiveness with the client. The therapist's own issues can and will affect how he or she views the client and the client's needs. The ability to separate our personal responses to the client, setting, process, music, and treatment team from the therapeutic relationship is essential to becoming an effective music therapist. The therapist's ability to utilize knowledge of self to enhance treatment and the therapeutic relationship is equally important.

Working with the Music

Music offers an almost limitless combination of possibilities in the therapeutic session. Music can be sung, played, and composed. Music can be a catalyst for movement, or it can be the focus of listening.

Bruscia (2014b) divides the possible uses of music into four methods: improvising, re-creating, composing, and receptive experiences. These categories, which offer a helpful way to begin thinking about the uses of music in therapy, are explored in later chapters of this book. It can also be helpful to begin to organize your own ideas about how to use music experiences in therapy. Record your ideas and those of your classmates in a notebook or electronic file. This will help to build your repertoire of available music experiences as you begin working with clients. Many of these experiences will be adaptable for use with different populations and will help to prime the pump of creativity when you need an idea to work with a group or an individual.

Bruscia (1998a) offers us a reminder that "although music therapy involves all levels of music experience, the closer the client's experience is to the purely musical level, the more certain we can be that it is truly music therapy" (p. 112). Begin now to accumulate musical experiences that will be useful to you and your clients as you work. We will address ways of working with the music in greater detail later in the book, including consideration of moving toward working from a music-centered perspective.

Assignments—Doing Music Therapy

Consider the following statements or questions as you begin to think about doing music therapy. You may find it helpful to do some journaling and discuss your ideas with your faculty supervisor.

- How do you know when you are healthy? Is being healthy different from being well?
- If you were a client in a session you observed or conducted, how would you have felt at various points in the session?
- Which definition of music therapy in this chapter do you agree with the most? Are there parts of the definition in which you are not in agreement or about which you are uncertain? Explain your answer.
- Can you describe a music experience that would fit the definition of music *as* therapy? Can you describe a music experience that would fit the definition of music *in* therapy?
- Describe an experience with music that helped you to understand something about the power of music as a therapeutic tool.
- Reflect on the importance of developing excellent music skills. Make a list of all the reasons you can think of that a music therapist needs to be a skilled musician.
- Listen to a piece of music that is appealing to you today. After listening, reflect on your personal responses to different timbres … dynamics … rhythms … tempos … lyrics.

2 Increasing Levels of Involvement

As explained in the Introduction, this book is arranged for future music therapists to use at various levels of their training. This chapter examines some of the experiences that students may have at each level of this process, including observing the music therapy session; participating and assisting as a student therapist; planning and co-leading; and, finally, leading the session. Since the tasks and challenges may be different at each level, this chapter is intended to help you understand and take advantage of those differences.

You may find research that has been conducted on aspects of what it is like to be a practicum student or intern useful in providing insights into issues that music therapy practicum students or interns find challenging. Wheeler (2002) interviewed practicum students about their experiences during music therapy practicums and found areas of concern and how they dealt with them. Wheeler and Williams (2012) focused on students' feelings about practicum supervision.

Other researchers have looked at areas of concern to interns. Madsen and Kaiser (1999) investigated the pre-internship fears of music therapy interns. Grant and McCarty (1990) examined emotional stages in the music therapy internship, while Knight (2008) compared ratings of pre-internship students and internship supervisors on items selected from the clinical foundations and music therapy categories of the AMTA *Professional Competencies* (American Music Therapy Association, 2013a). Finally, Clements-Cortes (2015) investigated perceptions of clinical, musical, and personal perceived skill development pre- and post-internship.

Although most of the contents of two books on music therapy supervision are focused on the supervisors, they can help music therapy students to gain insights into various aspects of the supervision process. They are *Music Therapy Supervision,* edited by Forinash (2001), and *Supervision of Music Therapy: A Theoretical and Practical Handbook,* edited by Odell-Miller and Richards (2009).

Observing the Session

Whether you are entering into the clinical world as an entry-level student or are further along in your education and training, you will undoubtedly encounter many new sights, sounds, feelings, and experiences. You will learn best if you allow yourself to experience all of these new stimuli and observe your own responses. You may develop your observation skills by trying this exercise: Imagine a room in your home or your dormitory room in your mind's eye. Write down as many details about the room as you can remember, then check your memory when you return to the room later. Another option: Look at a photograph or a drawing or painting for 30 seconds, studying the details. Cover the visual and write down as many details as you can before looking at the visual again to see how much you recall. A third exercise that may be useful involves simple, everyday items such as a pen, a book, a box of snacks, or other small items found in your environment. Place three items on a table and study them for 30 seconds. Turn away from the items and write down a description of what you saw—being careful to describe the details of the items. For example, don't write "a pen" but write "a long, cylindrical object, painted gray with white lettering along one side. At the end is a dark pink tip made of different material; at the opposite end is a sharp point of dark gray." This will help you learn to see details and hone your observation skills.

You may also want to explore more of these online at www.study-body-language.com/observation-exercise.html. This website includes many different types of exercises to train you to observe and remember what you see. You are encouraged to explore these exercises, especially Observation Exercise #3, Photographic Memory.

When you do your first observation (or on your first visit to a new site), consider the following elements that may influence your experience:

- The overall physical environment of the facility (location, size, age, etc.);
- The clients;
- The staff;
- The music therapist and the music therapy environment (variety of instruments and equipment, arrangement of room, etc.);
- The music therapy session structure (opening and closing, types of instruments and music used, techniques or interventions implemented, etc.);
- Your own reactions to the music therapy session.

In addition, consider the social and emotional environment from a client's perspective and as a staff member might be experiencing it. Also consider the client's response to you, to staff, and to the therapy process. Be especially aware of the following:

- Body language;
- Tone of voice;
- Arrangement of the therapy space;
- The sequence of events before, during, and after the therapy session;
- How the session ends;
- Where the clients return to when the session is over.

Pay attention to your reactions to different clinical populations. Are there settings in which you immediately feel a sense of connection and ease or, in contrast, in which you find yourself feeling uncomfortable and perhaps even disappointed or sad? Being open and honest with yourself and your advisors about your emotional response to different client populations is important and can provide you with opportunities to explore and resolve any unproductive or negative reactions, paving the way for more informed future placements. When you return from your observation experience, we strongly recommend that you write a journal or log entry about what you have experienced. You might use the elements listed above to help you or follow the format provided by your instructor or clinical supervisor. Abbott (2015) suggests a framework for making objective observations, including the time period in relation to the session (before, during, after), the constituents involved (who/what), and the type of involvement (musical or nonmusical).

Observing is a very important part of working in music therapy. If you are an entry-level student, you may even find that you are observing for most or all of a semester. Developing sharp observational skills will serve you well during your training and throughout your professional career.

Participating and Assisting

Once you have become familiar with a setting or have gained enough experience to be an active member of a therapy setting, you may be invited to participate in the therapy experience with the clients. Each therapist will have different ideas of how to integrate you into the session, but a few general guidelines may be helpful.

- Keep in mind that you are participating in the therapy of another. This session is not designed to address your needs, and, even if the process stirs up an issue that is real for you, you must edit your responses so that the focus of the therapy remains on the clients.
- Monitor your participation and keep your responses simple so as not to overshadow the client's responses.
- The therapist is the leader/facilitator of the session, and you must monitor your inclination to be helpful to clients or the therapist. Participation means just that— participate in the music experiences with the clients and be aware of your responses. Be acutely aware of the clients' responses as practice for your future role as therapist.

Participating in other therapists' sessions gives you a unique opportunity to learn about and gather music therapy interventions for later use in your own sessions. You also have the opportunity to observe your own responses to the many interventions that are used in music therapy. There is no substitute for personally experiencing processes that you will be asking a client to do when you are the leader of the session. Participate with constrained enthusiasm, offer encouragement to the clients as appropriate (the therapist in charge will guide you), learn all that you can about music interventions, and monitor and log your personal responses to the music experiences.

When it is time to assist with the session, you will have many options. Your supervising therapist may ask you to do specific things—for example, assist a client with holding and playing an instrument or support a child in successful group participation by assisting her to raise her hand to take a turn. At other times, what you are expected to do may be more open and left to your own judgment. In this case, you will need to monitor both your own and the client's behavior and responses to ensure that you are being helpful but not doing too much. In either case, your role as a helper is meant to do just that—help the client to get what he or she needs to get from the session.

Planning and Co-leading

You have now had an opportunity to observe the clients, to share in their experience of music therapy in this setting and possibly to assist, and to begin to understand the purposes of therapy for this client or group of clients. Now, focus your attention on the importance of planning and how it affects the outcome of co-leading a session.

Planning in therapy is a prerequisite for working with clients. You must have an idea of your goal or target in order to plan a map or route to get there. Once the goal or target has been defined, you might consider a number of routes, just as you would when choosing between going on a trip via the interstate highway or taking the scenic route. Deciding which route to take will depend on the responses of the clients to your interventions and on your current level of skill and knowledge. Even with the most thoughtful planning, you may discover that you begin traveling on one route but that client responses lead you to choose another route.

Whether you are working with another student or the music therapist at a clinical site, planning to co-lead a session requires clear communication about the intended destination, discussion of the options or routes to travel, and assignment of roles in this journey. Each therapist involved in the process must be prepared to ask questions of the other in order to clarify what will happen during the session—even when you are a student working with a professional. This discussion lays the groundwork for flexibility in dealing with unanticipated things that come up. For example, when the planning process has made it clear that Therapist A was thinking of using Song 1, but the final plan was determined to include Song 2, Song 1 remains an option if the client seems to need whatever Song 1 could offer. Therapist B can then invite Therapist A to insert Song 1 if it is appropriate to the needs of the client as the session unfolds. This level of cooperation provides clients with the best that both therapists have to offer.

Leading

Now that you have had the opportunity to observe and participate in music therapy sessions and to assist with, plan, and co-lead sessions, you are ready to take on the leadership of a session independently. You may experience a myriad of emotions as you plan to lead a session on your own for the first time. One person might be very excited and eager to put into action what has been learned, while another might find the prospect of being responsible for a client or group of clients anxiety-producing. It is normal to feel both of these emotions and many others. What you feel before leading a session independently is not as important as how you respond to your feelings. You will do better work if you acknowledge your emotional response to the task and prepare yourself to deal with the realities of your assignment. To increase your chances of successfully leading a session, try the following:

- Prepare by gathering information about your clients. This may be an assessment that you do yourself or may be based on information provided to you by the therapist or staff at your clinical site.
- Plan your session to achieve goals that are appropriate for your clients. Initially, use music and equipment with which you have skill and comfort.
- Don't be afraid to ask your professor or clinical supervisor for feedback, assistance, or support.
- Approach your first independent session with confidence; remember that you have something valuable to offer to your clients. Keep your focus on the needs of the clients and try not to focus on your own performance. This will go a long way in helping you to avoid the pitfalls of performance anxiety while working as a therapist.

Assignments—Increasing Levels of Involvement

These assignments can add to your understanding of each level of involvement in music therapy sessions:

- As soon as possible following a session observation, try to write down as much detail as you can recall. Think about creating a list of session elements, from the physical environment (e.g., the layout of the therapy room, what instruments were available, etc.) to the musical environment (what songs or genres of music were utilized, whether the music was all instrumental or vocal or a combination, whether the music was live or recorded or a combination, etc.), to the human element (how many clients were present, how the clients and instruments were positioned in the room, where the therapist was positioned in relation to the clients, etc.), to the session structure (how the session was opened and closed, the sorts of experiences that were implemented, how directive the therapist was, etc.). It is better to write too much than not enough. If possible, share this journal entry with the therapist you observed to see how comprehensive and accurate your recollections are.

- Using your journal or log, choose one personal response to an observation that stands out in your mind. This response may be positive or negative. Don't judge it, regardless of how you characterize it—just concentrate on trying to write and reflect on it in detail, describing it as fully as you can. What does this raise in your mind? What opportunities do you see?

- Reread a log entry about participating in a session with clients. Did you identify more with the clients or with the therapist? Was your energy focused more on how the clients were responding to the musical intervention, on what the therapist was doing, or on your own responses to the musical intervention? What can you learn about yourself as you reflect on what drew your attention the most? What might this say about your ability to separate your own issues from those of the clients when the music is happening? What will you do in the future to help you separate your issues from those of the clients?

- You are going to co-lead a session with the supervising therapist at your clinical site. Write out a strategy for how you will introduce, lead, and close a new experience for the client or group. Be careful to include ideas regarding how you will communicate with the supervising therapist (in this case, serving in the role as your co-therapist) to ensure that you include them in the experience while clarifying your role as leader.

- Think about a session that you recently led, using your journal or log to help you to remember the details, and choose something about the experience of leading that stands out in your mind. What was successful about your leadership? What could have been changed? How did you feel about being in this role? You will probably have other thoughts and feelings as you write about the session. Write about and reflect upon all of them.

3 Essential Aspects of Becoming a Music Therapist: Academic, Clinical Training, and Related Areas

As you move through your formal study of music therapy, your coursework will support and organize your growth and development through the sequencing of classes and experiential learning. From introductory classes to foundational music learning and history, to the development and application of clinical musicianship and therapy techniques culminating in your internship, you will be guided along a path of personal and professional growth. It is important for you to understand that the process of becoming a music therapist involves many facets. You will be expected to develop your identity as a clinical musician, as a therapist, as a healthcare professional, and as a member of the broader music therapy community. You are not expected to do this alone! Your faculty, advisors, and clinical supervisors are all available to help guide you on this journey. You will come to realize, over time, that it is the people with whom you work—your clients—who are the best teachers of what works in music therapy!

This chapter describes the essential aspects of becoming a music therapist in the United States. The differences in these specific aspects in various countries are so great that, in the opinion of the authors, it would be impossible to describe them for all countries. Therefore, professors and students in other countries will need to adapt it to what occurs in their countries.

Academic Preparation

The American Music Therapy Association, or AMTA (hereinafter referred to as "the Association" in this chapter), is the professional membership organization for music therapy in the United States. It lists the following as its goals:

1) To improve and advance the use of music, in both its breadth and quality, in medical, educational, and community settings for the betterment of the public health and welfare;
2) To serve as the primary organizational agency for music therapy professionals;
3) To develop, maintain, and seek continually to improve an organizational structure for the self-governance of the members of the music therapy profession.

The Association has established policies and standards that govern the education and training of music therapists, as well as guidance documents for professional music therapists. These include the *Code of Ethics* (American Music Therapy Association, 2014a); *Standards of Clinical Practice* (American Music Therapy Association, 2013b); and, in conjunction with the national certifying body, the Certification Board for Music Therapists, Inc. (CBMT), the *Scope of Music Therapy Practice* (American Music Therapy Association, 2015b; Certification Board for Music Therapists, 2015b). All of these documents as well as others are available on the Association website www.musictherapy.org and easily located by going to "Member Resources" and clicking on "Official Documents" and then the document itself.

All bachelor's- and master's-level music therapy degree programs in the United States are approved by the AMTA and accredited by the National Association of Schools of Music (NASM). While each academic program has its own unique qualities and may use differing terminology, the overall education and training of music therapists is standardized throughout the United States and is based on the AMTA *Standards for Education and Clinical Training*. These *Standards,* adopted by the Association in 2000, had undergone two revisions (2010, 2014) by the time of this writing. As with other Association documents referenced earlier in this chapter, the *Standards* are available on the Association website. For the convenience of the reader, we are including the main sections of the *Standards* here:

1.0   General Standards for Academic Programs
2.0   Standards for Competency-Based Education
3.0   Standards for Bachelor's Degrees
4.0   Standards for Master's Degrees
5.0   Standards for Doctoral Degrees
6.0   Standards for Qualifications and Staffing
7.0   Standards for Quality Assurance
8.0   Guidelines for Distance Learning

All approved academic study of music therapy in the United States is competency-based, with specific parameters identified for bachelor's, master's, and doctoral programs. Numerous resources are available on the Association website regarding education and training opportunities, and many of these are available even if you are not a member. Once on the website, click on "Education and Careers" and you will get a drop-down menu that includes the following selections:

- A Career in Music Therapy
- Schools Offering Music Therapy
- Education and Clinical Training Information
- National Roster Internship Sites
- Welcome to the Profession Intern Packets
- Advertise a Job in Music Therapy
- Find a Job in Music Therapy (available to members only)
- Scholarship Opportunities for AMTA Members
- Continuing Music Therapy Education

Bachelor's-Level Study

While the idea of master's-level entry to the field has been considered by practitioners for decades, the Association has undertaken the exploration of moving to master's-level entry to the field only since 2009, when the Education and Training Advisory Board (ETAB) proposed a retreat to more formally research and investigate such a transition. To learn more about the concept and the investigation into this thus far, you can visit the Association website, click on "Education and Careers," then on "Education and Clinical Training Information," and then on "Master's Level Entry Considerations" to access links for various documents and papers on this topic. The bachelor's degree remains the entry level for professional practice in the United States at the time of this writing.

The bachelor's degree is designed to address professional competencies outlined in the AMTA *Professional Competencies* (American Music Therapy Association, 2013a), with areas of study indicated by the Association in the *Standards for Education and Clinical Training* (American Music Therapy Association, 2014b) as falling into the following categories: musical foundations (45%), clinical foundations (15%), music therapy (15%, and including pre-internship and internship experiences), general education (20%–25%), and electives (5%).

Primary areas of study, including musical foundations, clinical foundations, and music therapy foundations and principles, are all further described in the AMTA *Professional Competencies*. The academic institution assumes responsibility for the creation and provision of coursework, providing guidance and oversight of the student's development, ensuring varied clinical training experiences and supporting the student to integrate coursework with practical skill development, and evaluating the student's progress at various points during their course of study to ensure competence before moving to the next level of study and practice.

Master's-Level Study

Master's degree programs are designed to impart greater depth and breadth of knowledge and skills in selected areas of the AMTA *Advanced Competencies,* with areas of study indicated by the Association in the *Standards for Education and Clinical Training* as falling into the categories of music therapy theory and advanced clinical skills, including supervisory skills. In addition, graduate study is intended to provide in-depth knowledge and competence in one or more of the following areas: research, musical development and personal growth, and clinical administration. Toward that end, programs design their curricular content and structure with varying foci, including some that are practice-oriented, others that are research-oriented, and still others that incorporate more of a blend of the two orientations. The *Advanced Competencies* document is the guiding resource for the development of master's degree programs, which serve to inform the creation of doctoral levels of study.

Doctoral-Level Study

Doctoral degree programs are intended to impart advanced competence from a much broader range of items in the AMTA *Advanced Competencies* document (American Music Therapy Association, 2015a) than a master's degree would cover. According to the *Standards for Education and Clinical Training,* doctoral programs "impart advanced competence in research, theory development, clinical practice, supervision, college teaching, and/or clinical administration, depending on the title and purpose of the program" (American Music Therapy Association, 2014b, n.p.). In 2016, there were eight doctoral degree programs in the United States.

Clinical Training

Different academic programs use different terminologies for the hands-on component of your education. For the purposes of this chapter, we will use the terminology from the *Standards,* "pre-internship" and "internship." These experiences occur on a continuum throughout your academic studies. Your practicum placements during your undergraduate coursework provide you with your first exposure to working with a variety of client populations (experience with at least three different populations is required) and with opportunities to work in both individual and group session formats, organized in such a way that you begin by observing, then move to participating and assisting, and then planning, co-leading, and, ultimately, leading.

Every student must complete a minimum of 1,200 hours of clinical training. Of these 1,200 hours, at least 15% (180 hours) must be completed in pre-internship experience and at least 75% (900 hours) in internship experiences. In addition to direct client contact, other experiences, such as supervision, session planning, and documentation, are required. These hours are minimums; additional hours may be required by faculty, by internship supervisors, or both, in order to ensure that the student has achieved the indicated competencies.

Pre-internship Training

Pre-internship training at one school may be referred to as "practicum," while another school refers to it as "fieldwork" and yet another school uses the term "clinical." Students are placed with music therapy supervisors in the community in a variety of settings. Additionally, in certain academic programs, opportunities for pre-internship training also occur at an on-campus clinic.

When approaching each new training site, you will want to learn as much as possible about the facility and the clients you will be seeing. Your site supervisor and your academic advisor can direct you to sources of information about the population that will help to prepare you for the experience. It is likely that each placement will have its own orientation to prepare you for working at the site. This orientation generally includes such information as what to do in the event of a fire drill, what you may or may not do as a student/volunteer, and what to do in the event of an injury or emergency. As a student in a clinical experience, you should not do anything that you have not been trained to do and should never do anything the site supervisor or orientation specifically describes as off-limits for students. Following the policies and procedures of the facility is an ethical responsibility.

Your academic advisor will provide you with a syllabus outlining the assignments, due dates, class topics, required readings, documentation responsibilities, and all the other information you will need to participate actively in this crucial part of your education and training.

Internship Training

Internship training can be designed in a variety of ways. There can be varying work schedules; it can be full- or part-time; it can occur at one facility or in several different settings; it can be near or distant from your school. Recognizing that many factors can be at play for each student pursuing their internship, there is flexibility built into the process.

At the time of this writing, there are two models of internship training approved by the Association: national roster and university-affiliated. Both types of training sites can operate under both models, that is, a national roster site can also accept university-affiliated interns and vice versa, as long as the therapist–intern ratios indicated in the *National Roster Internship Guidelines* are not compromised.

Regardless of whether the internship program is a national roster or university-affiliated site, the academic institution is responsible for developing an individualized training plan with each student. This training plan, based on the *Professional Competencies,* should take into account the individual student's entry-level skills in relation to the *Professional Competencies* as well as the student's needs and life circumstances. Clinical training supervisors collaborate with the academic faculty to implement the individualized training plan and support each intern in achieving the competencies. The individualized training plan should also indicate the number of pre-internship hours already completed by the student and the remaining internship hours required, along with outlining requirements such as the roles and responsibilities of the student, the qualified on-site supervisor, and the academic faculty. A written internship agreement is also established between the student, internship supervisor, and academic faculty, outlining the entry and exit competencies for the student. The internship agreement may also include other information such as the length of the internship, the intern's work schedule, the supervision plan, and agency-specific requirements such as background checks, liability insurance, etc. For more information on these latter areas, please see the section later in this chapter on Related Responsibilities.

National Roster Internships

National roster internship sites undergo a rigorous review and approval process through the AMTA Association Internship Approval Committee (AIAC). The *National Roster Internship Guidelines* document outlines the general requirements for a site to be approved as a national roster site (including eligibility of the setting, ratio of therapists to interns, policies and procedures for supervision and evaluation of interns, and the requirements and responsibilities of the supervising therapist[s] and internship director, as well as the responsibilities of interns and academic faculty). Once approved as a national roster internship site, there is ongoing communication and oversight between the internship site and the AIAC, as the national roster site is responsible for updating the committee on all changes at the site in addition to submitting a final site evaluation which must be completed by all interns at the conclusion of their training. As of September 2016, there were 194 approved national roster sites listed on the Association website.

University-Affiliated Internships

Rather than being approved and reviewed by the AIAC, university-affiliated internships are reviewed by the Academic Program Approval Committee (APAC) as part of each school's academic program approval or reapproval process. University-affiliated internships must meet all Association standards for clinical training but are arranged directly by academic faculty in consultation and collaboration with area therapists. Students participating in a university-affiliated internship must be under the direct supervision of an on-site credentialed music therapist for at least half of their internship hours. If the on-site supervisor is unavailable, the student must be under the direct supervision of a credentialed music therapist under the auspices of the university.

Related Responsibilities

As you progress through your clinical training experiences, both pre-internship and internship, you will find that there are many responsibilities inherent in being a healthcare professional. While this book seeks to provide you with materials and resources to support your development as a clinician, it is important that you also recognize and understand the importance of other responsibilities expected of all people working in settings in which you may find yourself serving clients.

Both pre-internship and internship experiences are opportunities for you to practice professional behavior. Professionals demonstrate responsibility by (a) attending as scheduled, (b) communicating any changes in plans, (c) dressing appropriately for the setting, (d) being prepared for the session, (e) documenting according to site policies, (f) protecting client confidentiality and privacy, (g) maintaining appropriate boundaries, (h) cooperating with staff, and (i) being open to feedback and supervision. These topics are likely to be discussed by your academic advisor, your site supervisor, and your clinical training director. You will hear this information repeatedly because your behavior as a professional reflects on the field of music therapy and how others perceive it.

During pre-internship and internship training opportunities, you may be required to undergo or report on a variety of health and legal reviews as well as fulfill certain training requirements beyond your music therapy training. For example, it is commonplace for pre-internship students and interns to be required to provide medical information such as a vaccination history, to undergo testing for tuberculosis (this test is called a PPD test), and to receive a vaccine for hepatitis B. Background checks, including fingerprinting, are fairly routine for internship placements. With regard to training requirements, Infection Control, Cybersecurity, and the Health Insurance Portability and Accountability Act (HIPAA) are typical requirements at many healthcare facilities.

Supervision

Participating in supervision is critical to your development as a music therapist. It can be the difference between achieving your own personal and professional goals and missing the mark. Music therapy supervision takes many forms: It can be individual or group; it can be formal or informal; it can include observation and feedback; it may involve the sharing of specific concepts and hands-on training; it can be provided in writing or verbally; it can incorporate the use of audio and video materials for viewing and listening, as well as recording your own work for documentation and feedback; it may include preparatory assignments, including journaling, assigned readings, focused listening, and practicing; and it can include the use of music.

While supervision is a requirement of your pre-internship and internship experiences, it is important also to understand and appreciate the essential role that it can play in your ongoing development after you enter the professional workplace. As therapists, we pride ourselves on our ability to create and nurture relationships, specifically relationships that support and motivate our clients to move toward health. Supervision is just such a relationship, but in a professional realm rather than a clinical one. As Forinash (2001) stated, "The focus of the supervision relationship is to address the complexities involved in helping supervisees in their ongoing (and never-ending) development as competent and compassionate professionals. Supervision is a relationship, one in which both supervisor and supervisee actively participate and interact" (p. 1).

As you can see, the process of supervision is an active and dynamic one that demands your participation; it is not a lecture that you attend (although processing a lecture with your supervisor could be a valuable undertaking!), but a shared commitment between yourself and your supervisor. Different supervisors will have different styles, so it is up to you, the supervisee, to advocate for yourself to ensure that you are getting what you need from supervision. Come prepared with questions, concerns, and ideas!

In addition to supporting you in areas such as developing strategies for session work, improving your professional writing skills, practicing techniques for working with difficult clients, and other sorts of "work" duties, other outcomes of music therapy supervision are related to the development of your identity as a music therapist. Identity is defined as "the qualities, beliefs, etc., that make a particular person or group different from others" ("Identity," 2016). As a profession, music therapy is still a young discipline, so our group identity continues to evolve as our theory, research, and practice develop. Bruscia (2014b) addresses the identity of our profession extensively. As an individual, you are just starting to develop your identity as a music therapist. In a conference presentation (1984), Bruscia suggested that there were several important factors in developing an identity as a music therapist, but that the single most important pursuit is this: to understand your clients through their music. Supervision plays a pivotal role in this.

Closely related to developing your identity as a music therapist is your development as an ethical practitioner. Ethics are much more than the AMTA *Code of Ethics* document. Dileo (2000) has dedicated an entire book to the topic, and you are encouraged to review her work.

Finally, effective supervision, in combination with experiences in your clinical work, may lead you to a point at which the need or desire for more personal work becomes evident. Gardstrom and Jackson (2011) explored this question in a survey of AMTA academic program coordinators. The survey asked about three specific types of therapy—verbal therapy, music therapy, and expressive arts therapy other than music therapy—and sought to determine whether any of these were required or encouraged. Although undergoing personal therapy is not currently a component of the Association *Standards for Education and Clinical Training*, results of the survey indicated a broad range of perspectives and implementation among music therapy faculty. Some programs require students to pursue personal therapy, some programs strongly encourage it, and some programs do not specifically address it as part of their curriculum.

Dileo (2000) addresses topics of personal and professional competence as well as professional self-care for music therapists and speaks to the important contributions that personal therapy and supervision can provide.

Bruscia (2014b) makes a direct connection between ethical practice and competence with his concept of reflexivity, as well as ensuring that we, as music therapists, maintain our own unique relationship to music and use it to nurture ourselves, reminding us to hold on to the joy of music in our own lives.

Remember what brought you here: the music!

Important Documents

As mentioned earlier in this chapter in the section on Academic Preparation, there are numerous documents regarding education and clinical training, as well as other topics, available on the Association website (www.musictherapy.org), and you are encouraged to access these and familiarize yourself with the information.

In addition to the supportive materials available through the Association, there are other documents of great importance to you as you work to achieve your professional credential, MT-BC (Music Therapist-Board Certified). The Certification Board for Music Therapists, Inc. (CBMT) website (www.cbmt.org) contains information regarding examination, certification, advocacy, and more. All of the information and procedures related to applying for and taking the CBMT examination are outlined on the website, and you may find that you are interested in purchasing the self-assessment examination (SAE) to help prepare yourself for the actual certification exam. In addition to examination and certification information, the CBMT website also includes the *Code of Professional Practice,* to which all certificants must adhere, along with information related to advocacy and state recognition.

Finally, AMTA offers scholarships for students and interns, as well as a *Welcome to the Professional World* packet to support you as you transition from your role as a student to that of being a professional. You can request this packet at the midterm point of your internship; the form and requirements are all available on the Association website.

Assignments—Essential Aspects of Becoming a Music Therapist

These exercises will serve to guide you in becoming more familiar with the AMTA and CBMT websites and with various documents related to your education and clinical training, as well as to support you in considering the importance of being an active participant in supervision:

- Go to www.musictherapy.org and find the AMTA *Code of Ethics* and *Professional Competencies* documents. Review the "Preamble" in the *Code of Ethics* and then compare it with section B.9, Clinical Foundations—The Therapeutic Relationship, in the *Professional Competencies* document. Consider how these two sections relate and how they support your work in music therapy.
- Go to www.musictherapy.org and find the *Advisory on Levels of Practice in Music Therapy* document. Read the section titled "Professional Level of Practice." For each of the four sections described (Professional Growth, Musical Development, Personal Development of the Therapist, and Clinical Experience), reflect on your own level of achievement at this time. Identify skills and abilities with which you feel confident and competent; based on this, try to determine some short- and long-term goals for yourself, including strategies for achieving them. Discuss these ideas with your faculty advisor to see how your self-perceptions align with the perspectives of your advisor.
- Go to www.cbmt.org and find the section titled "Preparing for the Exam." Review the *Board Certification Domains* document. How do these align with the AMTA *Professional Competencies?* How can you use both of these documents to help support and guide you as you move through your education and clinical training experiences and ultimately prepare to sit for the certification exam?
- When you are about halfway through your internship, go on the CBMT website. In the "Preparing for the Exam" section, review the "Exam Candidate Handbook." Prepare any questions you have about applying for, preparing for, and taking the examination. Bring these questions to a meeting with your internship supervisor and ask for their guidance. You may also want to discuss the possibility of taking the Self-Assessment Exam (SAE) as part of your preparation for seeking board certification.
- When you are at the midterm point of your internship, go on the AMTA website. In the "Education and Careers" section, find the "Welcome to the Profession Intern Packets" link. Read about this benefit, download and complete the form, and bring it with you to a meeting with your internship supervisor for their signature.

4 The Process of Planning for Music Therapy

There are a number of things to consider as you begin to plan the content and sequence of a session. All of these, of course, are aimed at developing a session that is most productive and beneficial for your clients. The result will be a session in which the goals are appropriate to meet the needs of your clients and the procedures that you use are both appropriate to the goals for the clients and congruent with your values, skills, and knowledge.

Before exploring personal beliefs and values, though, it is important to have a context for understanding the client. Underlying all work in therapy is a sense of who the client is, why he or she has entered a therapy relationship, and what the outcome of that therapy is intended to be.

The Client's Perspective

What Is Important to the Client?

It is very important to keep in mind that our clients are, first and foremost, people. No matter how many challenges or diagnoses they have or how many restrictions on their functioning, they are unique, complex, evolving human beings. Maslow (1999) emphasizes the importance of reminding ourselves that we must view each client as the unique individual they are and not simply as a member of a group. There are some questions that we might ask about the person with whom we are working and things that we may discover that will help us to treat him or her as an individual. You may want to think about the following:

- *What does he or she like to do?* Consider the kinds of things your client enjoys doing and/or is good at doing, with whom he or she enjoys doing these things, and where these things are done.
- *What does he or she not like to do?* Consider the things the client does not like to do, resists doing, or may find boring, frustrating, or undesirable.
- *What would he or she like to change?* Consider what the client dislikes about him- or herself, finds to be unproductive about his or her personal behavior, experiences as obstacles to living life to its fullest, and would like to change.
- *What does he or she picture for life in the future?* Consider what he or she wants from life, what image he or she has for the future, and what hopes or desires he or she has for life.
- *How can we help to make these things happen?* Consider the supports that he or she has; the supports that he or she needs; which, if any, of these supports music therapy can provide; the methods that can be used to provide them; and what could compromise his or her safety, participation, or success and thus should be avoided.

In answering each of these questions, think about the following: What do you see, hear, observe, sense, or understand that leads you to these answers?

What Can the Client Gain from Music Therapy?

While the questions in the above section are important and help us to see our client as a person, we also need to be aware of what the person needs to function better and to be healthier—in other words, why he or she was referred to treatment and to music therapy. You can learn a lot by noticing on an intuitive level what he or she communicates while you are talking or playing music together or what you observe that he or she needs in order to function more fully or to be healthier.

The process of assessing the client for music therapy is more complex than simply responding to these considerations, and it is important to remember that music therapy cannot help with all problems. But your initial observations will give you an intuitive sense of how you might be able to help the person.

The Music Therapist's Perspective
How Do I Feel About the Client?

It is important to become aware of our own feelings as we begin our work in music therapy. Our feelings form the basis of how we relate to our clients and show us where we need to work to improve our ability to relate to people. As music therapists, we may work with people who have various types of life or health circumstances or disabilities. It is helpful for us to be aware of our feelings toward people who find themselves in any of these circumstances. Each of these reactions can give us information about our underlying attitudes and beliefs about what it means to be *healthy* and *normal.*

It can be helpful to examine how we feel when we see a person with a disability. For example, we may feel uncomfortable. We may want to reach out to help the person or we may shy away, perhaps out of fear of not saying or doing the right thing. We may find ourselves turning away from someone with a particular disability or avoiding eye contact. Some people feel uncomfortable when a person with a physical disability is struggling to cross the street. If you have ever had the experience of offering to help a person in this position but been told that he or she did not need help, think of how you felt.

You may have listened to someone who stutters trying to say a word and not known if you should try to help the person find the word or just wait. Think about how you felt at this time. If you have ever encountered a person who was exhibiting mental health difficulties in the community, think of how you reacted and felt. If you have been involved with people who are dealing with a terminal illness, it will be helpful to consider what your feelings were during this process. Maybe you were uncomfortable with the dying process or perhaps you feel that you came to a better understanding and acceptance of it during that time.

It may be helpful also to think about how you feel when people you know have encountered difficulties. Perhaps a friend has had to deal with a life-threatening illness or a family lost their home and had to go to a shelter. Think of how you responded to this kind of situation. Think about how you feel when you watch a television movie about a painful life event, whether you identify with the person struggling or with those who come to the aid of that individual. This may tell you something about your personal attraction to the helping professions.

We may have many reactions when dealing with people with disabilities and challenges. It is not possible to say whether our reactions are right or wrong, normal or abnormal. However, we can use our awareness of them to help us understand our feelings about people who are different from us or who are encountering difficult situations and to grow from our awareness. This is an important part of becoming a therapist. As Maslow (1999) said, "Only the one who respects health can do therapy" (p. 61).

What Is My Personal Theory of Helping?

An important influence on a music therapist's work is what may be called a *personal theory of helping*. The development of such a theory will help the therapist in many ways. You will develop your own theory based on your beliefs about various aspects of the helping process. It ultimately becomes a reflection of who you are and how you see the world and the place of therapy within this world. This theory serves as a guide for making decisions as part of the therapy process. It will be revised over time as you mature and your views change.

Considering the potentials and limitations of what it means to help may be useful as you develop your personal theory of helping. Bruscia (2014b) provides a framework of ideas that can organize and guide your efforts as you reflect on this. He begins by clarifying the significance of two main points: first, the limitations inherent in doing therapy (not just music therapy, but all forms of therapy), and second, the value of understanding the unique characteristics of how music therapy helps.

First, in reference to the limitations that both therapists and clients must confront throughout the process of therapy, Bruscia (2014b) reminds us that the therapist can only help and cannot actually make the changes—only the client can do that. Maslow (1999) supports this approach:

> We can't *force* him to grow, we can only *coax* him to, make it more possible for him, in the trust that simply experiencing the new experience will make him prefer it. *Only* he can prefer it; no one can prefer it for him. If it is to become part of him, *he* must like it. If he doesn't, we must gracefully concede that it is not for him at this moment. (p. 62)

Second, Bruscia (2014b) goes on to clarify that, in music therapy, help occurs as a result of both the client's interaction and relationship with *the therapist* and their interaction and relationship with *the music*. In your role as therapist, it is your responsibility to develop a deep understanding of each client with whom you work. Based on this understanding, you will be able to determine how to best support the client and facilitate their growth forward toward health.

Bruscia (2014b) then details a comprehensive overview of ways of helping that are unique to music therapy. In considering the following, you may think that this list could apply to any form of therapy, and, at first glance, you would seem to be correct. However, these ways of helping are defined and described as musical processes:

- "Being there" for the client,
- Understanding the client's needs and resources,
- Empathizing with the client,
- Giving voice to the client,
- Interacting with the client,
- Holding and anchoring,
- Communicating with the client,
- Providing opportunities for self-reflection,
- Presenting and exploring alternatives,
- Guiding as necessary,
- Connecting the client to self and world,

- Providing redress,
- Intervening when necessary,
- Motivating,
- Validating and affirming,
- Caring for the client,
- Protecting one's own ability to help. (pp. 75–90)

As you can see, the simple act of providing therapy is not so simple! As a caring and compassionate music therapist, you must dedicate the time and energy to developing and maintaining your clinical musicianship and your own health in order to be fully present in service to your clients. Your theory of helping may also embrace the philosophy embodied in one or more psychotherapeutic frameworks or be part of a framework based on an indigenous model of music therapy.

Many books are available to give more information on aspects of becoming a helper. We recommend *The Helping Relationship: Process and Skills*, 8th edition, by Brammer and MacDonald; *Becoming a Helper*, 7th edition, by Corey and Corey (2015); and *Intentional Interviewing and Counseling: Facilitating Client Development in a Multicultural Society*, 8th edition, by Ivey, Ivey, and Zalaquett (2014).

How Do I Find Music Helpful?

Since the tool that we use in music therapy is music, it is also helpful to explore our own relationship with music. Think about how you use music in your own life. Perhaps you turn on recorded music when you get home, or maybe you play live music. Consider your purpose in doing so. Maybe it serves to help you relax and relieve stress, or perhaps you find that it gives you energy. Think about the types of music you choose for listening or playing at various times and in different situations and how you are using music to meet your own needs. You might also consider what instruments you use to make music. How do you choose? Is it the timbre or other qualities of the sound, the range of pitches available, the means of playing (breath vs. striking a percussion instrument), your level of comfort or technical skill, or some other quality?

There are obviously many ways for us to use music, and it will be helpful to explore these in our own lives. You might also think of times when you have felt uncomfortable listening to music and what may have elicited this discomfort. Your exploration of the place music holds in your own life will give you insights as you consider how you can help your clients use music in their lives. Dedicate some time and consideration to this. In addition to reflecting and journaling on these ideas, we recommend seeking out others' perspectives on this. Some recommended resources include *The Music Within You*, 2nd edition, by Katsh and Merle-Fishman (1998); *Moving to Higher Ground: How Jazz Can Change Your Life*, by Marsalis (2008); and *The Music Lesson*, by Wooten (2006). Seek out others on your own!

Ethical Considerations

Each of us has ethical standards that we follow in our personal lives. Of course, these may vary from person to person. There are ethical as well as legal standards that govern our societies, although there is also room for variation in some of these areas.

It is helpful to explore our personal ethical standards. Begin by asking yourself how you decide whether what you are doing is right or wrong. Do you look to an external source (such as formal religion) or to what your parents taught you? You have probably internalized much of what you have been taught so that you may not consciously think about the source but rather do what comes naturally. Have you ever done something, then felt that it was not right and gone back and made amends or changed it? What process led to this decision? Consider whether you judge others as doing things that are right or wrong and, if you do, whether it ever occurs to you that their values or ethical standards may be different from yours but not necessarily wrong. Consider how you would determine for certain if they were wrong or right, or whether this determination can even be made.

Reflecting on these issues is the beginning of developing skill in ethical thinking. Since ethical dilemmas occur in all areas of our lives, it is helpful to begin thinking about how each of us defines our boundaries between ethical and unethical, right and wrong.

All therapists are confronted with ethical situations that test our personal and professional boundaries, ask us to choose between two or more difficult paths of action, and force us to choose the action that will do the least harm to a client in a given situation. The process we use for making these decisions is a result of how we were raised, our life experiences, and the amount of time that we have devoted to reflecting on how we might respond to ethical dilemmas.

It is important to be aware of the code of ethics of the professional organization in one's country. For U.S. music therapists, this is the AMTA *Code of Ethics* (American Music Therapy Association, 2014a); U.S. music therapists should also be aware of the CBMT *Code of Professional Practice* (Certification Board for Music Therapists, 2011). *Ethical Thinking in Music Therapy* by Dileo (2000) is an invaluable resource for considering ethical issues in music therapy. *Issues and Ethics in the Helping Professions,* 9ᵗʰ edition, by Corey, Corey, Corey, and Callanan (2014), is a classic text that applies to ethical issues in the helping professions beyond music therapy.

Assignments—The Process of Planning for Music Therapy

Consider the following to provide insights on planning for therapy:

- A number of questions were asked under "What Is Important to the Client?" Think of a client you are working with or have worked with or observed in the past and reflect on these questions and issues in relation to this individual. After considering this and notating your thoughts, apply the same questions to yourself. In doing so, do you feel that you are better prepared to empathize with a broader range of individuals you may meet in your work?
- Consider your reactions as discussed under "How Do I Feel About the Client?" Spend some time journaling about your feelings as related to the problems and issues discussed.
- Begin to develop your personal theory of helping. Consider the limitations identified in the section on "What Is My Personal Theory of Helping?"—that the therapist can only help and cannot actually make the changes for the client (nor force the client to make the changes). How can you begin to develop your clinical musicianship and clinical facilitation skills, based on the processes listed? Developing a personal theory of helping is not an easy process, but as you write and reflect and revise, it will come together over time. Refer back to this as you continue to develop as a music therapist and expect that it will continue to change and grow as you do.

- Discuss some of your own responses to music as raised under "How Do I Find Music Helpful?" Can you identify times when you feel that all you need is music? Are there other times when you feel that you need something more? What would that be?
- Think of an ethical issue specifically related to clinical work with which you have been confronted. If you have not yet experienced such a situation, you may want to refer to some of the "Additional Learning Experiences" found throughout Dileo's *Ethical Thinking in Music Therapy* (2000) as a resource for examples. Reflect on your decision-making process, including where you sought guidance, and write up a summary of the process and the outcome. What will you take from this experience to help prepare yourself for future challenging situations?

5 Client Assessment

Assessment is a multistep process involving gathering information, observing the client, interpreting the client's responses to music and to the therapist and other clients, and using this information to plan for treatment. Assessment involves information gathering, in a session or sessions, to more fully understand the client's strengths and needs, interests, and preferences. Assessment also includes information gathered from client records and from others involved in the client's care, such as family care givers, direct care workers, and professional staff. Analysis of assessment data leads to a determination of the suitability of music therapy treatment for a particular client and may help to identify treatment approaches or strategies. Decisions about assessment approaches and tools are dependent upon the theoretical orientation of the music therapist, the policies of a setting, the characteristics of a population group, and the tools available for assessing that group.

The element that distinguishes music therapy assessment from other types of assessment, such as educational or psychological assessment, is that the assessment typically occurs while a client is engaged in a music experience, usually improvising, performing or re-creating, composing, or listening to music.

Any type of music therapy assessment involves observing the client making or listening to music under specific musical conditions that enable the therapist to assess the client's abilities and needs. In so doing, the therapist draws conclusions about the client that influence the client's music therapy in some way. The purposes of assessment are varied and may include (a) prescription, (b) diagnosis, (c) interpretation, (d) description, and (e) evaluation (Bruscia, 1993, 2003).

Another element of assessment is that information about the client, both musical and nonmusical, can be gathered in a variety of ways. Sometimes, the therapist briefly interviews the client and, based upon this interview, decides how the music therapy session will unfold, usually within the same session. This may be the case in medical settings, in which the therapist may meet the patient only once and the purpose of therapy is to manage the patient's symptoms. In other kinds of assessments, the therapist engages the client in very specific sequences of musical activities and records the client's ability to complete the tasks presented. This is quite often the case in educational settings, where music therapists are interested in assessing a client's skills in order to develop a music therapy treatment plan as part of the Individualized Education Plan (IEP). Consequently, the degree of organization and formality also varies considerably in music therapy assessments. In some situations, the assessment phase is limited to a brief verbal interview to determine the nature of the client's immediate problems or concerns and musical preferences. This is usually followed by the music therapist engaging the client in a musical experience with a goal in mind while continuing to assess the client. In other situations, the client's assessment is formalized, with the client and therapist meeting for a specific period of time to conduct the assessment; only after the assessment is completed, interpreted, and placed in a written form does the client move into the treatment phase of therapy, and only if this is indicated by the findings of the assessment.

The final element of an assessment to be considered is the manner in which the assessment is documented and presented to others. In some situations, the therapist is the only one who deals with the assessment. For example, in a medical setting, where assessment and treatment can occur within the same session, the therapist may record only a brief written description of the goals and outcomes of the session in the patient's chart, without any broader discussion of the patient with other staff members. In other situations, the assessment of the client may lead to a detailed written report that is shared with or discussed with others. This may include the client him- or herself, the client's family, or the clinical team. There are many variations in the manner in which the music therapy assessment can be communicated to others; this largely appears to depend on the setting in which the music therapist works and his or her role in the treatment team.

Guidance and expectations for assessment are included in the AMTA *Standards of Clinical Practice* (American Music Therapy Association, 2013b). They include the general categories of functioning to be assessed, the appropriateness of methods used, and other aspects to consider in assessing a client. The standards specify that the assessment procedures and results will become a part of the client's file and that the "results, conclusions, and implications of the music therapy assessment will become the basis for the client's music therapy program and will be communicated to others involved with provision of services to the client. When appropriate, the results will be communicated to the client." It is a good idea to refer to these assessment standards while learning and doing assessments, as they provide guidance for planning, implementing, and reporting music therapy assessments (General Standards, 2.0). The *Board Certification Domains* of the Certification Board for Music Therapists (CBMT) (2015a) identify components of assessment, interpretation, and reporting common to music therapy practice and expected of certificants.

In summary, music therapy assessment usually involves:

- Observing the client making or listening to music under specific musical conditions that enable the therapist to assess the client's abilities, needs, and interests;
- One or more of the following purposes: diagnosis, prescription, interpretation, description, evaluation (Bruscia, 1993, 2003);
- Varying degrees of complexity. In some situations, it may be limited to a brief interview, while in others it may involve an extended period of engagement and observation;
- Variations in the ways in which the assessment is recorded and communicated to others.

More information about the use of assessment in music therapy is available in the book chapters Music Therapy Assessment (Wheeler, 2013) in Feder's *The Art and Science of Evaluation in the Arts Therapies,* 2nd edition, and Music Therapy Assessment (Lipe, 2015) in *Music Therapy Handbook.*

Why *Music Therapy* Assessment?

It is only through *music therapy* assessment that we can know the strengths and needs of the music therapy client. This has a twofold advantage. First, it enables the music therapist to observe and interpret the ways in which the client uses musical media and consequently identify treatment goals from within the musical media themselves. Second, it allows the therapist to make some determination about the actual music therapy experiences that will be most beneficial for the client. In order to meet the goals of therapy, should the client be improvising, performing or re-creating, composing, or listening to music? Should the sessions be structured, semistructured, or created spontaneously according to how the client presents at the beginning of the session? These questions can be explored and are often answered as an outcome of the assessment process. So, in music therapy assessment, the outcomes of assessment are not just a determination of the treatment goals but also the musical modality (e.g., improvising, writing songs, participating in musical activities) that best facilitates these goals. In addition, the music therapy assessment can give the therapist guidance as to the subsequent structure and sequence of sessions (to the extent that predicting a session sequence is possible and desirable). Assessment data may also provide a baseline for use in evaluating changes in client response over time.

There are also other benefits to undertaking a music therapy assessment with a client. Clients may perform differently in music than in other modalities (Bruscia, 1988; Coleman & Brunk, 2003). For example, children with autism or Rett syndrome may engage in or respond to musical activities in ways that are different from activities that are verbally based. This in turn may provide insight into the child's skills and strengths that were not previously evident. Older adults, especially those with cognitive deficits, may respond in the presence of music when they have been unresponsive in other settings (Keough, King, & Lemmerman, 2016). Additionally, some service providers require a music therapy assessment and treatment plan in order to justify the provision of music therapy or for reimbursement purposes (Scalenghe & Murphy, 2000). Finally, a clinician cannot ethically provide services to a client without making some assessment of the client's needs and the kinds of interventions that are appropriate in meeting these needs.

The Process of Assessment

Receiving a Referral

The process of assessing a client often begins with a referral. A referral is a request by a staff member or agency to see the client for music therapy, although in some situations clients will refer themselves or the referral may come from a family member. The referral may be made because the client is experiencing a symptom that can be addressed by a music therapist (such as presurgical anxiety) or because the overall goals of treatment can be addressed in music therapy (such as a drug rehabilitation program). The purpose of assessing the client is to determine his or her suitability for music therapy. It is often the responsibility of the music therapist to establish criteria and a system for referral. Ghetti and Hannan (2008) provide an example of referral criteria for a pediatric intensive care unit and note that this also provides an avenue to educate others involved in a client's care to the potential benefits of music therapy.

Gathering Background Information

Almost every assessment involves gathering background information on the client. This can take various forms, including one or more of the following:

1) Reading the client's chart or file,
2) Interviewing the client,
3) Interviewing family members,
4) Discussing the client with staff members.

Typically, the purpose of gathering this background information is to gain (a) an understanding of the person; (b) knowledge of major events in the person's life and their impact; (c) medical conditions and medications taken; (d) an understanding of the types of programs (educational, therapeutic, etc.) in which the person has been involved, if any, and the outcomes of these programs; (e) an understanding of the client's relationship with music, previous music experiences, and so forth; (f) awareness of his or her spiritual or religious values and beliefs; and (g) knowledge of the current needs and goals. Depending on the setting, it may also be necessary to learn about therapeutic *methods* undertaken with the client. For example, in some settings, behavioral interventions, reward systems, or specific forms of consequences (e.g., time out) may be utilized with the client, and it may be necessary for the music therapist to understand these interventions and incorporate them into sessions. This will depend largely upon the philosophy of the setting and the personal philosophy of the music therapist.

The breadth and depth of information on the client varies considerably with each stage of the assessment process. In some situations, such as those in which you expect to see the client for an extended period of time (as is often the case in a school or residential setting), you will garner a comprehensive understanding of the client's history, needs, and goals. In other situations, such as when you meet with the client only once, you will gather only the information necessary for addressing the client's immediate needs. Regardless of the extent to which you gather background information, you need to build an understanding of the client that helps you contextualize your music therapy assessment and subsequent goals of treatment.

Determining the Purpose and Type of Assessment

The next stage in the assessment process, determining the purpose and type of assessment, is by far the most complex and difficult to understand because of the number of variables that need to be considered in selecting and completing a music therapy assessment.

The first element that needs to be considered is the *overall purpose* of the assessment. As previously mentioned, there are five main purposes in assessing a client in music therapy that have been defined by Bruscia (1993, 2003): diagnosis, interpretation, description, prescription, and evaluation. These will be discussed in some detail below.

A second element to consider is the *domains* (Bruscia, 2003) of the assessment, which Bruscia defines as "those aspects or facets of the human being that the music therapist is trying to understand" (personal communication, April 12, 2005). For example, do you want to understand how much arm movement a client with cerebral palsy has while playing the drum, or do you wish to understand the music listening preferences of an adult with late-stage cancer? The first question involves assessing the physical skills or abilities of the client, whereas the second question involves assessing the music preferences of the client. Bruscia (1993, 2003) has identified various domain areas related to music therapy assessment. The *Board Certification Domains* (Certification Board for Music Therapists, 2015a) target cognitive, communicative, emotional, musical, physiological, psychosocial, sensorimotor, and spiritual domains for assessment, along with biographical and medical information.

The third element to consider is the *sources of musical information* (Bruscia, 1993). As we discussed earlier, from what types of musical experiences do we need to be gathering the assessment data? Should the client be improvising, performing or re-creating, composing, or listening to music? Each of these ways of creating and experiencing music allows you to gather different kinds of information on the client.

In summary, you need to consider the following when undertaking an assessment:

- The overall purpose of the assessment: diagnosis, interpretation, description, prescription, evaluation;
- The domains: biographical, somatic, behavioral, skill, personality or sense of self, affective, and interactional;

- The sources of musical information: improvising, performing or re-creating, composing, or listening to music.

Overall Purpose of the Assessment

As stated above, the purpose of the assessment may be diagnostic, interpretive, descriptive, prescriptive, or evaluative. It is common for assessments to have more than one purpose. Thus, an assessment may be both descriptive and evaluative or both interpretive and prescriptive, and so on.

Diagnostic Assessment

The first general focus of assessment is *diagnostic*. As the word implies, diagnostic assessments are concerned with efforts to "detect, define, explain, and classify the client's pathology, focusing primarily on its causes, symptoms, severity, and prognosis" (Bruscia, 1993, p. 5). When music therapy assessments are diagnostic in nature, musical criteria are used to determine whether the client has a condition, to determine the type of condition the client has, or to determine how the client experiences or perceives the condition. It is important to distinguish the purposes of diagnostic assessments by music therapists, or of music therapists gathering diagnostic information, from diagnostic work that is done by professionals in some other disciplines. Music therapists are not allowed by law to *diagnose;* diagnosis is the purview of some other disciplines whose training and scope of practice includes diagnosis. Thus, the information that a music therapist can discover about a client that can be used in diagnosis can be used to understand the client and may assist those who are charged with making a formal diagnosis. Within these boundaries, it should be understood that the information that a music therapist can provide through a diagnostic assessment can be uniquely discovered through music therapy and can perform a valuable function in understanding the client.

The MATADOC (Music Therapy Assessment Tool for Awareness in Disorders of Consciousness) has been researched over many years and is robust when compared to similar validated measures currently used to diagnose awareness in persons with disorders of consciousness (Magee, Siegert, Daveson, Lenton-Smith, & Taylor, 2014; Magee, Siegert, Taylor, Daveson, & Lenton-Smith, 2016). Validity has been established with MATADOC for use with adults only; research continues to explore its validity with children with disorders of consciousness (Magee, Ghetti, & Moyer, 2015) and its clinical utility with adults with end-stage dementia (W. Magee, personal communication, September 12, 2016).

Interpretive Assessment

The second general focus of assessment is *interpretive,* in which "efforts are made to explain the client's problems in terms of a particular theory, construct, or body of knowledge" (Bruscia, 1988, p. 5). The first step in doing an interpretive assessment is to gather samples of the client's music-making or responses to music, and the second step is to make inferences about these responses with reference to the chosen construct or theory. The assessment may be designed according to a particular theory or may be a general inventory that allows interpretation according to a variety of theories, depending on which is most relevant to the client's responses.

Examples of interpretive assessments include an assessment by Rider (1981) in which he sought to discover if the ages at which children could perform musical tasks that involved increasingly complex levels of cognitive functioning correlated with the difficulty of the tasks. His framework was the developmental theory of Piaget, and the musical tasks were modeled after nonmusical tasks used by Piaget. Since Rider's assessment sought to explain the children in terms of Piaget's theory, this assessment qualifies as an interpretive assessment.

Another example of an interpretive assessment comes from Priestley's (1975, 1994) work in Analytical Music Therapy (see also Scheiby, 2015). Priestley's work was grounded in the psychoanalytic constructs of Freud, Klein, and Jung, wherein she would interpret the musical improvisations of her clients according to relevant constructs, such as defense mechanisms, ego, id, superego, and drives.

Descriptive Assessment

The third focus of assessment is *descriptive,* in which efforts are made to understand the client and the client's world in reference only to him- or herself (Bruscia, 1993). In descriptive music therapy assessments, the client's musical experiences are meaningful in and of themselves and in relation to other facets of the client's life.

Scalenghe and Murphy (2000) provide a sample music therapy assessment for managed care that is descriptive (pp. 28–29). This assessment is divided into nine major areas: history of present illness, behavioral observations, motor skills, communication skills, cognitive skills, auditory perceptual skills, social skills, specific musical behaviors, and summary and recommendations. In this assessment, typical of descriptive assessments, the client is thoroughly described in terms of his or her skills and needs, with a summary and recommendations oriented toward identifying the goals of treatment.

Chlan and Heiderscheit (2009) developed the music assessment tool (MAT) to be used in intensive care units with mechanically ventilated patients. Because of severe communication problems, it is important to have a means of gathering music preference and experience information in order to select music to benefit these patients. The tool utilizes yes/no questions along with some demographic and current medical condition information to guide the music therapist and/or nurses in choosing music for use with the patient.

Prescriptive Assessment

The fourth focus of assessment is *prescriptive,* intended to determine the treatment needs of the client and to provide a database for formulating goals, placing the client in the appropriate programs, and identifying the most effective methods of treatment (Bruscia, 1993, p. 5). Prescriptive assessments have multiple purposes, for example, determining:

- Whether music therapy is needed and whether the client wants music therapy;
- Whether there are any contraindications for participating in music therapy;
- Which methods of music therapy are most suitable (e.g., improvising, listening to, creating music);
- The kinds of materials that are appropriate for the client's age, maturity, and interests;
- Whether the client has the prerequisites for participating in existing music therapy programs.

In all cases, these questions require comparing what the client needs and wants to what music therapy can provide.

The Special Education Music Therapy Assessment Process (SEMTAP, Brunk & Coleman, 2000; Coleman & Brunk, 2003) is an example of a prescriptive assessment. This assessment compares the child's performance on musical and nonmusical tasks that are part of the Individual Education Program (IEP) goals and objectives or the goals that have been set for the child's education. This assessment meets the criteria of a prescriptive assessment because it (a) attempts to determine whether music therapy is indicated for a child, and (b) suggests those musical activities which will best meet the child's IEP goals.

Carpente (2013) developed a process designed to assess musical-play interactions with individuals with neurodevelopmental disorders (IMCAP-ND). Consisting of three scales (musical–social–emotional capacity, musical cognitive, and perception and musical responsiveness), this assessment seeks to evaluate the client's developmental ability to perceive, interpret, and engage in interactive music-making. The data are used to guide the therapist in planning treatment.

Evaluative Assessment

The fifth focus of assessment is *evaluative,* wherein the purpose is to establish a basis for determining progress. These types of assessments are concerned with gathering data on the client prior to beginning music therapy and then using these data as a baseline for determining the effects of treatment.

As an example of an evaluative assessment, McDermott, Orrell, and Ridder (2015) developed the Music in Dementia Assessment Scales (MiDAS), a series of five visual analog scales to measure the responses of persons with dementia in music therapy groups. According to Chase (2002), one purpose of an evaluative assessment is to "document the positive impact of music therapy" (p. 25) by using the results of the initial assessment as a baseline from which to measure changes in the children's abilities as a result of music therapy. Carpente (2013) states that the IMCAP-ND is also designed to be used for pre- and post-treatment measurement, thus indicating progress.

Domains of Assessment

Although these general purposes of assessment give you guidelines about where to focus your attention with the client (i.e., diagnosis, interpretation, etc.), you now need to consider the specific goals of your assessment. In the section that follows, you will be introduced to various *domains* (Bruscia, 2003) of assessment in music therapy. Each domain has its own specific character and focus. Further, as you become familiar with the various types of music therapy assessments, you will begin to see that some assessments focus comprehensively on only one domain (e.g., Bonny, 1980, Music Experience Questionnaire), while others contain elements of multiple domain areas (e.g., Coleman & Brunk, 2003, SEMTAP).

Biographical

This domain is concerned with gathering background information on the client, as outlined earlier in this chapter. This includes a broad range of information on the client from a variety of sources—his or her family, education, interests, important life experiences, relationship to music, medications, clinical diagnoses, previous experiences in therapy, and so forth. Although gathering biographical information often occurs prior to undertaking a music therapy assessment, it can sometimes occur within the assessment itself. When this occurs, formal guidelines can be given for gathering information (e.g., Coleman & Brunk, 2003), or it can be gathered in an open-ended interview (e.g., Priestley, 1994).

Somatic

This domain is concerned with gathering information about the client's physiological and psychophysiological responses to music (Bruscia, 2003). This includes physical responses to music-making and listening, such as measurements of heart rate, respiration, blood pressure, EEG, and EMG. Additionally, it includes psychophysiological responses to music-making and listening, such as pain perception, consciousness, tension, fatigue, and anxiety, among a vast range of measures (Bruscia, 2003).

When gathering somatic information, music therapists are often concerned with the effects of a music experience (typically, listening to or performing music) on one or more aspects of a person's physiology or psychophysiology. For example, Wigram (1997) assessed the effects of vibroacoustic therapy (Skille, 1997) on arousal levels, hedonic tone, blood pressure, pulse rate, and mood prior to, during, and after treatment using a variety of mechanical (such as a blood pressure monitor) and self-report measures (UWIST Mood Adjective Check List; Matthews, Jones, & Chamberlain, 1990).

As this domain might suggest, assessments in this area are quite often not unique to music therapy. For example, Sandrock and James (1989) reviewed assessment instruments used to measure various psychophysiological responses to music and identified 10 distinct inventories, scales, and checklists, none of which had been designed by a music therapist.

Behavioral

This domain deals with the client's observable behaviors. According to Bruscia (1993):

> Behavioral assessment is the process of observing and analyzing what the client does or how the client conducts him-/herself. This includes overt action, reaction to stimulation, or interaction with the environment that can be seen, heard, or otherwise noted by the therapist. Behaviors may be assessed in isolation, in reference to their stimulus or reinforcement conditions, or as an integral part of their interpersonal and environmental contexts. (p. 43)

Bruscia (1993) suggests that four main approaches to behavioral assessment have been undertaken in music therapy: (a) measuring clearly defined isolated behaviors (e.g., eye contact) and using these measures as a baseline for determining the effects of treatment; (b) charting the behavioral interactions between clients (e.g., number of times one client touches another inappropriately); (c) rating clients according to their tendencies to exhibit behaviors or behavioral categories in a specially designed inventory (e.g., number of times the client followed the directions of the therapist in a session); and (d) recording entire sequences of behaviors and then analyzing them according to content, sequence, or structure (e.g., while a client performs in a group instrumental piece).

A number of music therapists have developed assessments that focus on clients' behavior. These include Bitcon (2000), Boxill (1985), and Merle-Fishman and Marcus (1982) for children and Hanser (1999) for general use.

The General Behavior Checklist, developed by Bruscia (1993) and shown in Table 5.1, considers broad areas of client behavior and responses in the areas of (a) motivation, (b) nonverbal interaction, (c) communication skills, (d) relationships, (e) adaptive behaviors, (f) aggressiveness, (g) energy, (h) physical capabilities, (i) reality orientation, and (j) motor deviances. This inventory serves "as a guide for observing and recording whether or not the client exhibits each of the behaviors listed" (p. 54).

Other methods for behavioral assessment (Bruscia, 1993) include (a) *measuring targeted behaviors,* in which specific behaviors are examined in detail, assessing the conditions under which they occur; (b) *measuring interactive behaviors,* in which the therapist examines how the behavior of one person affects or is influenced by the behavior of another; and (c) *documenting a behavior stream,* which involves recording a wide range of behaviors sequentially within a specific time period (e.g., the first 5 minutes of a session).

Skill

This domain entails a broad range of musical and nonmusical skills demonstrated by the client (Bruscia, 2003), including (a) sensorimotor skills involved in music-making and listening (gross motor, fine motor, visual motor, reflexes, coordination, postural, etc.); (b) perceptual motor skills involved in music-making and listening (perception of figure–ground and part–whole relationships, visual and auditory discrimination skills, etc.); and (c) cognitive skills involved in music-making and listening (attending skills; short- and long-term recall; choice-making; basic academics such as colors, numbers, reading, writing, and telling time; size discrimination; spatial relationships; sequencing; problem-solving; cause and effect; modes of response and learning styles; etc.). The skill domain also includes creative abilities (the client's capacity for creating and responding to music) and musical skills (technical music-making; ability to read music, match pitch, imitate rhythm, etc.).

Table 5.1
General Behavior Checklist (Bruscia, 1993)
Used with permission.

Motivation
Attends sessions
Participates
Works toward goals
Nonverbal Interaction
Eye contact
Physical contact
Musical contact
Communication Skills
Understands language
Speaks
Signs/gestures
Reads and writes
Relationships
Interacts with therapist
Relates positively to therapist
Interacts with other clients
Relates positively to other clients
Takes leader role in group
Takes follower role in group
Works toward group goal
Adaptive Behavior
Stays in room
Stays in seat
Attends

Aggressiveness
Screams/tantrums
Verbally attacks therapist
Verbally attacks other clients
Physically attacks therapist
Physically attacks other clients
Destroys property
Energy
Hyperactive/hypoactive
Impulsive/reflective
Fast-moving/slow-moving
Tired/energetic
Physical Capabilities
Walks independently
Uses arms and hands
Has tremors or spasms
Vision loss
Hearing loss
Seizures
Toilets self
Reality Orientation
Temporal orientation
Spatial orientation
Sense of identity
Short-term memory

Behaves relevantly
Follows rules
Goes along with wishes of others
Waits for turn
Handles materials responsibly
Shares materials with others
Behaves safely

Long-term memory
Hallucinations/delusions
Relevance of behavior
Motor Deviances
Rocking
Tapping
Perseverative movements
Stereotypic finger/hand movements
Stereotypic head movements
Stereotypic arm movements
Twirling
Tics
Grimacing

Liberatore and Layman (1999) developed the Cleveland Music Therapy Assessment of Infants and Toddlers to assess the skills of infants and toddlers who were at risk. Their assessment scales are divided into distinct developmental time periods (such as 0–3 months, 3–5 months) and identify specific skills within each period according to (a) cognitive skills, (b) gross motor skills, and (c) fine motor skills. The assessment procedure requires the music therapist to design activities in which these skills can be observed and assessed.

Numerous other skill assessments have been developed, including Nordoff and Robbins's (1971) Categories of Response. Sabbatella and Lazo (2015) designed the Music Therapy Assessment Protocol for assessing the sound–musical development of children, ages 3-6 years, diagnosed with developmental disorders.

Personality or Sense of Self

This domain involves gathering information on the psychological nature of one's *self,* including (a) self-awareness, (b) self-esteem, (c) identity formation, and (d) unconscious aspects of personality (Bruscia, 1993). Personality assessments also fall within this category (e.g., Cattell & Anderson, 1953).

The vast majority of assessments in music therapy focused on one's sense of self have been projective in nature, and many of these have their origins outside music therapy. *Projective assessments* are based upon the premise that clients can *project* conscious and unconscious aspects of themselves onto or into musical materials. This can include interpreting sounds or music, rating musical excerpts while listening to them, or improvising music on various *givens,* such as playing a family member or emotion.

Several projective assessments have been developed, all of which use recorded music or sounds to elicit responses from listeners (Ball & Bernardoni, 1953; Braverman & Chevigny, 1964; Bruscia & Maranto, 1985; Husni-Palacios & Palacios, 1964; Shakow & Rosenzweig, 1940; Van den Daele, 1967; Wilmer & Husni, 1953). In some situations, musical excerpts are used (e.g., Van den Daele, 1967), whereas in others (e.g., Wilmer & Husni, 1953) distorted or nonmusical sounds (e.g., a train) are used. In some of these assessments, the listener or client is asked to write down whatever comes to mind after listening to the sound, while in others he or she is asked to narrate a story while the music plays. Various forms of analysis have been developed, including content analysis, structural analysis, and the interpretation of the client's responses according to a theory or construct (e.g., Freud's theory of psychosexual development or Piaget's theory of cognitive development).

Emerging from his clinical experiences with both adults and children, Bruscia (1987) developed the Improvisation Assessment Profiles (IAPs), "designed to provide a comprehensive method for assessing client[s] through an analysis and interpretation of their musical improvisations" (Bruscia, 1993, p. 84). The IAPs involve three interrelated procedural stages, which usually take several sessions to complete: (a) clinical observations of the client improvising under a variety of musical and interpersonal conditions, (b) musical analysis of the improvisations, and (c) interpretation of the data. While Bruscia describes the main assessment domains of the IAPs as emotional and interpersonal (1993), this method of assessment has been placed within the personality or sense of self domain because of the comprehensive intra- and interpersonal nature of the assessment process and the fact that the interpretive levels of the IAPs involve examining both conscious and unconscious aspects of the person and their implications for therapeutic goals and treatment.

Affective

This domain involves gathering information on the ways in which a client responds emotionally while listening to music or expresses him- or herself emotionally when making music. It also involves the preferences clients have for listening to music.

In order to map out the emotional responses of clients to improvising music in Analytical Music Therapy, Priestley (1994) developed The Emotional Spectrum, consisting of the following main emotions: freeze–fear, flight–fear, defensive fear, anger, guilt, sorrow, love, joy, and peace. Priestley asked her clients to create improvisations on each of these emotions and then played back the improvisations to the clients, asking them for their reactions. In this way, a rich battery of information was gathered about clients' emotional expressions while making music and their associations with these emotions.

While Nordoff and Robbins's (1971) Categories of Response look at the musical skills of the child, they are simultaneously concerned with the ways in which the child responds to the mood or changes of mood in the music. Thus, the assessment process is concerned with understanding the child in both musical and emotional terms.

Baxter, Berghofer, MacEwan, Nelson, Peters, and Roberts (2007) created an assessment instrument using therapist-created music experiences for use with children and adolescents with multiple disabilities. They measure emotional responses in the Individualized Music Therapy Assessment Profiles (IMTAP) and specifically assess range and appropriateness of affect, emotional expression, and regulation.

Various other assessment scales are concerned with understanding how a person responds emotionally while listening to or performing music (Hoffren, 1964; Robazza, Macaluso, & D'Urso, 1994; Steinberg & Raith, 1985). For example, Asmus (1985) developed a nine-element rating scale for the measurement of affective responses while listening to music, finding that over 75% of raters used the following dimensions of affect when rating the pieces: evil, sensual, potent, humorous, pastoral, longing, depression, sedative, and activity.

Interactional

Ultimately, music-making in therapy is a shared experience, even if it is just one therapist and one client making music together. The interactional domain is primarily concerned with the following four interactional dimensions (Bruscia, 2003): (a) communicativeness—the extent to which the client communicates with others; (b) the client–therapist relationship; (c) peer relationships and group skills in music therapy; and (d) family relationships.

Interactional assessments have been approached in a variety of ways (Goodman, 1989;

Hough, 1982; Pavlicevic & Trevarthen, 1989). Broucek (1987) developed an interactional assessment based upon the theory of Harry Stack Sullivan. She drew parallels between musical interactions and designated interpersonal behaviors, suggesting that disturbed behavior would be manifest in musical interactions. By assessing these interactions, the therapist could develop an understanding of the client's problems and how these could be resolved musically. Pavlicevic and Trevarthen (1989) took a similar approach to assessing the joint musical improvisations of clients with schizophrenia and depression. They were primarily interested in the diagnostic potential of analyzing their clients' improvisations in order to determine whether there were any differences in the levels of musical contact of adults with differing psychiatric diagnoses. To meet this goal, they developed the Index of Music Experience and the Music Improvisation Rating Scale.

Based on earlier work (Jacobsen, 2012; Jacobsen & Wigram, 2007), Jacobsen and McKinney (2015) demonstrated the reliability and validity of the use of the APC-R (Assessment of Parenting Competencies-Revised), a musical improvisation assessment tool designed to assess affect attunement, early nonverbal communication between parent and infant, and parental emotional response. This assessment is designed to contribute to child protection decisions.

In addition to the Categories of Response discussed in the domains of skill assessment and affective assessment, Nordoff and Robbins (2007) also developed three additional evaluation scales that can be viewed as primarily interactional in nature, although the affective and skill components are also apparent. Scale 1, The Child-Therapist Relationship in Coactive Musical Experience, is a seven-level scale that looks at levels of participation and qualities of resistiveness. Scale 2, Musical Communicativeness, also a seven-level scale, assesses levels of communicativeness through three modes of response (instrumental, vocal, and body movement). Scale 3 is called Musicing: Forms of Activity, Stages, and Qualities of Engagement. This is by far the most comprehensive and complex of the rating scales and incorporates areas of rating through instrumental coactivity, including basic beat tempo range, rhythmic forms, and expressive components, as well as singing and melodic forms.

Sources of Musical Information

As is already apparent, the same musical experiences used to assess clients for music therapy are used in music therapy treatment: improvising, performing or re-creating, composing, and listening (Bruscia, 1993). Each kind of music experience offers a different way of gathering information about the client. For example, listening assessments are primarily concerned with gathering information about the ways in which a client hears, receives, or reacts to sound (Bruscia), whereas improvisational assessments are primarily concerned with the ways in which "the client extemporaneously makes up music or creates expressive sound forms while singing or playing" (Bruscia, p. 16). Notice that the first has to do with *receiving* the music, while the latter is concerned with *creating and receiving* the music simultaneously. This, in turn, has implications for the type of assessment information you want to gather about the client. Do you want to understand how a client perceives or takes in something or how he or she creates something? Thus, the musical media themselves are important because of the nature of the tasks and challenges contained within each experience.

Improvising Assessments

When improvising is used as the vehicle for assessment, the therapist is concerned with the ways in which the client creates music while playing or singing. Improvisational assessments can be concerned with solo, duet, or ensemble playing, referentially or nonreferentially, and with or without lyrics. Improvising is also well suited for projective assessment because the ways in which "the person creates and produces his/her own music extemporaneously—to meet musical and interpersonal demands given in the here-and-now—is a manifestation of how the person relates to self and others at conscious and unconscious levels" (Bruscia, 1993, p. 16).

Improvisational assessments are particularly appropriate for people who have trouble expressing themselves verbally, for those with identity and self-awareness issues, for those with interpersonal and communication problems, and for those who lack spontaneity (Bruscia, 1993). Loewy (2000) describes an improvisation assessment for use in music psychotherapy wherein the therapist gains an understanding of the client through expression and interaction in music-making.

Performing or Re-creating Assessments

Performing or re-creating assessments are concerned with assessing the ways in which the "client learns or performs vocal or instrumental music or reproduces any kind of sound form or musical pattern presented as a model" (Bruscia, 1993, p. 13). According to Bruscia, there are three primary media: vocal, instrumental, and movement. In vocal experiences, the client is engaged in a variety of tasks that focus on the ways in which he or she uses his or her voice, imitates sounds and melodies, learns songs, sings from notation, sings in an ensemble, and so on. Instrumental experiences are concerned with the ways in which the client manipulates instruments; imitates sounds, rhythms, and melodies on instruments; learns precomposed pieces; plays in ensemble; reads from notation; and so forth. Movement experiences are concerned with the ways in which the client uses his or her body and performs rhythmic body tasks, sequences of movements, movement dramatizations, and so on.

Re-creative assessments are particularly well suited to assessing within the skill domain because the therapist has the opportunity to observe a range of skills as they are contained with each re-creative experience (e.g., vocal or instrumental motor skills, rhythmic skills, tonal skills). Bruscia (1993) identifies two main objectives to skills assessments: (a) to identify a developmental delay or disability; and (b) to identify loss of function due to organic injury or disease, delay, or disability. A third objective in skills assessment is the identification of baseline knowledge and abilities that may serve as evaluative measures in treatment.

Composing Assessments

Composing (or creative) assessments are concerned with examining the ways in which the client composes a song or instrumental piece, usually with the help of the therapist. Herein, the therapist may be interested in how the client creates and organizes the composition (skill domain). These experiences are appropriate for projective assessments. They are useful for people who have problems focusing on a task, making decisions, and taking responsibility for them; problems in organizing and sequencing ideas; and a need for documenting inner feelings or achievements (Bruscia, 1993). Composing may also be an effective assessment style for clients who have difficulty in using verbal interaction but who may be able to share thoughts and feelings in songs or instrumental music forms.

Listening Assessments

Listening or receptive experiences are those in which the client hears, receives, or reacts in some way to an auditory stimulus, which may be music or any of its components. The music may be live or recorded and of any type. The client may be asked to respond verbally or nonverbally (Bruscia, 1993). Listening assessments address a broad range of domains. For example, in projective listening assessments (Cattell & McMichael, 1960; Mazzagati, 1975; Van den Daele, 1967), the client responds to music and sounds affectively, for the purposes of understanding conscious and unconscious aspects of the person's personality. Listening assessments can also be used for the somatic domain, where the therapist observes the physiological and psychophysiological responses to music, or in the skill domain, where the therapist is concerned with the receptive skills of the client (e.g., ability to apprehend the sound, distinguish sounds). The Computer-Based Music Perception Assessment for Children (CMPAC) (Wolfe, Waldon, & Bilbe, 2006, as cited in Wolfe & Waldon, 2009) is designed to assess children's musical preferences using a laptop computer and preprogrammed musical genres/selections. The Music Attentiveness Screening Assessment (MASA) (Wolfe & Waldon, 2009) is used to assess a child's ability to focus attention for a period of time during a music listening task. The authors suggest that these two tools can be used as part of the assessment process to help make decisions about which children will respond well to music therapy.

According to Bruscia (2003), listening assessments are indicated for clients who need to (a) be activated or soothed physically or emotionally, (b) learn how to listen, (c) examine their own feelings and ideas, (d) reminisce, and (e) have spiritual experiences.

Conducting the Assessment

Once you have established the overall purpose, domains, and sources of musical information for your assessment, several procedural steps follow naturally: (a) gathering the data, (b) summarizing and/or interpreting the findings, and (c) reporting the findings.

As you prepare for each assessment, it is important to consider the practicalities of conducting an assessment. Two main elements should be considered: space and time. Ideally, find a physical space that allows uninterrupted privacy with a minimum of extraneous noise. Additionally, make sure that this room is of adequate size and contains all the musical materials you will need to complete the assessment. Sometimes these can be set out in advance (Wigram, 2000a), whereas in other situations you will need to present to the client only those instruments that are needed for each task.

Wherever possible, choose a time of day that gives the client his or her best opportunity of responding to the assessment tasks (Liberatore & Layman, 1999). Sometimes it may be necessary to conduct an entire assessment in smaller blocks of time because the client is not able to manage the entire assessment in one sitting.

Gathering the Data

You can begin to see that there are many ways to gather data about the client. Gathering data, which refers to the actual way in which you collect information about the client, is different than sources of musical information, which refers to the type of musical experience from which you observe the client. Bruscia (2003) has identified the following methods of gathering data:

1) *Record survey:* Gathering information from written sources such as files and charts.
2) *Tasks and activities:* Gathering information by observing the ways in which the client completes various tasks and activities.
3) *Verbal inquiry:* Interviews, in-therapy conversations, and questionnaires.
4) *Observations:* Observing the way the client conducts him- or herself in and

sometimes outside music therapy.

5) *Tests:* Objective and projective tests.

6) *Physical measurements:* Heart rate, blood pressure, and so forth, measured by machines.

7) *Analysis of materials:* Analyzing musical materials such as improvisations; interpreting these according to specific theories or constructs.

8) *Indirect methods:* Interviewing family, staff members, and so on.

9) Notice that different assessment needs suggest different methods of gathering data. For example, if a music therapist is interested in assessing the effect of music listening on blood pressure, heart rate, and stress levels, then he or she is likely to use physical measures and tests. If, however, the music therapist is interested in the levels of interaction between the client and therapist, then he or she is likely to analyze the musical materials of the session.

Summarizing and/or Interpreting the Findings

Once you have collected your data, you need to summarize and/or interpret these findings. In some assessments, this involves collating and summarizing scores or ratings or indicating whether a skill or behavior is present or absent. Examples include Bruscia's (1993) General Behavior Checklist (see Table 5.1) and Liberatore and Layman's (1999) Cleveland Music Therapy Assessment, both of which require the therapist to indicate whether certain behaviors or skills are present or absent.

Taking a different approach, Priestley (1994) developed the Patient Questionnaire for use in Analytical Music Therapy. This assessment is used to gather descriptive information on the client at the beginning of therapy. Priestley developed categories of questions around various aspects of the biographical domain, such as family history, musical history, present psychological condition, goals, and spiritual life. Responses to each of these areas are written down by the therapist, and this information can then be combined with other sources of information, such as the Emotional Spectrum and interpretations of the client's improvisations, to gain an overall psychological picture of the client. Loewy (2000) emphasizes the importance of using language to convey the meaning in the music created in the assessment process.

Taking yet another approach, Shultis (1995) developed the Music Therapy Assessment and Initial Treatment Plan (see Table 5.2) to assess clients in medical settings. Her assessment covers several different domains, including biographical (diagnosis, medical history, musical history, current therapies) and behavioral (presenting affective state), and then provides sections through which the goals and types of music therapy interventions are indicated. Note that this format is easily adapted to a computerized patient record or electronic health record with the list of responses in each category expanded to allow for quick selection of those items that best describe the client. All sections include an option for "other" to allow for unstated information and objectives to be added.

Table 5.2
Music Therapy Assessment and Initial Treatment Plan (Shultis, 1995)
Used with permission.

Patient information: diagnosis, length of stay at referral, reason for referral, referral source, previous hospitalizations/treatment, and level of orientation
Support systems: family/friends/living arrangements
Current problems: things such as pain control, sleep disturbance, nutritional deficiencies, breathing difficulties, anxiety, depression, anger, acting out, agitation, noncompliance, confusion, need for palliative care; and treatments or therapies (include medications for pain, anxiety, depression, psychosis, sleep)
Musical history/preferences:
Observations made during assessment: for example, does the client exhibit anxiety; is he or she talkative, unresponsive, and so forth?
Treatment assignment: individual sessions and frequency versus group assignment and schedule
Goal areas for treatment: areas such as anxiety, depression, pain management, coping skills; also indicate treatment team goals for this patient
Treatment interventions: (indicate all that were used in gathering data and the client's responses)

___ singing	___ leisure/music skills building	___ lyric writing
___ musical games	___ composition of music	___ lyric analysis
___ improvisation	___ playing instruments	___ music as nonverbal communication
___ imagery for relaxation	___ imagery for self exploration	
___ patient-selected music	___ other _____	
___ for self-expression		
___ for independent listening		
___ relaxation training/techniques		

Objectives for treatment: As a result of these interventions, the patient	**Target date**	**Short Form for charting**
___ will demonstrate a decrease in symptoms of anxiety	by	(↓ anxiety)

Additional objectives in the assessment address patient needs related to agitation, breathing, cognition, coping skills, depression, nonverbal communication, pain, post-discharge resource access, relaxation skills, self-expression, and verbal response level.

This example is a truncated form. The original includes multiple prestated objectives along with spaces for additional objectives as needed for individual patient needs.

Reporting the Findings

The final procedural step involves reporting the findings to others. In some clinical situations, the report is given to other team members, while in others, it is communicated verbally during a team or family meeting. The findings may also be shared with third-party payers or with parents of children in treatment. In yet other situations, only the music therapist or members of the music therapy department see the report. The choice of to whom the findings are communicated depends largely on the setting in which the music therapist works and the specific goals of the assessment. Of course, these are merely guidelines to help you think about reporting the findings and to help you understand that they can be reported in a wide variety of ways. It is essential that music therapists follow HIPAA (Health Insurance Portability and Accountability Act) regulations when sharing client information with others. A primary purpose of this law is to make it easier for people to keep health insurance. Additional outcomes include protecting the confidentiality and security of healthcare information (which is increasingly maintained electronically) and helping to control administrative costs in the healthcare industry.

If Music Therapy Is Not Recommended

Almost every music therapy assessment requires the therapist to ask a basic question: Is music therapy recommended for the client? In some assessment situations, this is easily answered: The client may not be responsive to music, may not be engaged or interested in the music therapy strategies, or may not respond in a way that is sufficiently different from other, nonmusical therapies (such as speech therapy) to warrant inclusion in a music therapy program. However, to examine this question thoughtfully, several factors warrant consideration.

While a client may not be responsive during the music therapy assessment, this does not necessarily mean that he or she is not suitable for music therapy. In some clinical situations, nonresponsiveness may be the therapeutic issue presented by the client, so that the music therapist is able to observe and assess the ways in which the client is nonresponsive, how this is performed musically, how nonresponsiveness sounds, and the various associated nonmusical behaviors. The purpose of assessing the client may be to describe (descriptive assessment) the client, with a focus on his or her nonresponsiveness or to interpret (interpretive assessment) the nonresponsiveness according to a theory or construct (e.g., that nonresponsiveness is a form of resistance that could be understood in a larger psychological way). The MATADOC assessment was developed specifically to assess responsiveness in people who are minimally responsive and have complex problems. This means, for example, that their ability or will to respond might be masked by complex physical difficulties, making even a tiny physical gesture impossible. It is therefore important to measure responsiveness carefully across a number of domains (e.g., physical, communication). This assessment provides a protocol to document minimal responses that might be missed by less sensitive measures (Magee et al., 2014).

Similarly, while resistance, agitation, avoidance, or even aggression may be indicators that music therapy is not recommended, these same behaviors can also be the very reason the client was referred to music therapy. For example, a client with Alzheimer's disease may be referred to music therapy because of increased agitation and aggressiveness toward others. The purpose of the assessment process may be to observe the client's aggressiveness and agitation in music therapy and examine the ways in which various musical interventions mediate, reduce, or otherwise change the client's behavior.

Assessing the suitability of a client for music therapy is therefore context-bound. In some clinical situations, the behaviors and responses of a client may be indicators that the client is not suitable for music therapy, whereas in others, these same behaviors may be manifestations of the client's therapeutic issues, which can then be observed and assessed within various kinds of music experiences (sources of musical information).

Issues in Music Therapy Assessment

Before we move into examining several music therapy assessments in detail, let us briefly examine some of the current issues in music therapy assessment.

Taking a Quantitative or Qualitative Approach

The first issue for consideration is the extent to which your assessment needs to be approached from a quantitative or a qualitative perspective (Bruscia, 1993).

For our purposes, we may think of a *quantitative assessment* as when the music therapist is interested in gathering information about various aspects of the client's behavior or condition and attempting to do this using numbers, inventories, or other methods that provide a numerical measure of the person's skill, attribute, or response. For example, Liberatore and Layman's (1999) Cleveland Music Therapy Assessment is a quantitative assessment because the music therapist rates (using yes or no) the extent to which a particular skill or behavior is present. Based upon a tally of skills, the music therapist can determine the developmental level of the client and the extent to which music therapy is indicated for that person.

A *qualitative assessment* is more concerned with describing the ways in which clients respond to or work with various music experiences. This may also include interpreting the client's music-making according to nonmusical theories or constructs. Many biographical assessments are qualitative because the information gathered is descriptive and cannot be reduced to numerical values. An example of a qualitative assessment is Bruscia's (1987) Improvisational Assessment Profiles (IAPs), which are based upon interpreting the music improvisations of clients according to several interrelated procedural steps.

When it is important to know how well or how much a client performs or whether he or she has certain kinds of skills, behaviors, or characteristics, then a quantitative assessment is likely to be indicated. For example, when measuring physiological responses to music, it is likely that the music therapist will want to know how high the client's client blood pressure is, what his or her heart rate is, and how much this changes while listening to music. If, however, the therapist wishes to know how the client feels while listening to his or her own improvisation or that of a parent or partner, then the music therapist is more likely to want to do this qualitatively.

Reliability and Validity Issues

A second issue concerns the reliability and validity of music therapy assessments. This issue has not been adequately addressed in music therapy assessment, even though it has previously been raised (Bruscia, 1988). Reliability and validity are associated only with quantitative assessments. "Reliability" refers to the extent to which the data collected are free from measurement errors (Meadows, 2000). That is, do the data accurately represent the phenomenon observed, or are they distorted, misrepresented, or incompletely recorded? "Validity" refers to the extent to which the assessment measures the construct under investigation and is an "indication of its utility and meaningfulness in clinical and research situations" (Meadows, p. 9).

For example, Meadows conducted a validity study on the Guided Imagery and Responsiveness Scale (GIMR) developed by Bruscia (2000). Bruscia argued that responsiveness to the Guided Imagery and Music experience was an indication of psychological health and that scores on the GIMR should therefore be positively related to other measures of health and negatively related to measures of psychological defensiveness. In order to assess the validity of the GIMR, a series of studies was conducted to examine the relationships between scores on the GIMR and two measures of psychological health. While such studies are important in the development of assessments in music therapy, little is being done to evaluate the reliability and validity assessment measures.

Another ongoing issue in music therapy assessment is the extent to which assessments need to be norm-referenced or criterion-referenced (Coleman & Brunk, 1997). Very few music therapy assessments are norm-referenced. As described above, norm-referenced assessments allow comparison to some known group. Large numbers of people are tested with the tool in order to get data for norm-referenced assessments. Information is then provided as to how various portions of the group scored on the assessment. This information can then be used to compare the performance of an individual or group to the larger group that was tested. There are some areas, particularly those in which music therapy assessments are used for diagnostic purposes, in which norm-referenced assessment data would be strongly indicated, allowing comparisons of the performance of a client that one music therapist assesses with others who have similar diagnoses or characteristics. Since many tests in psychology are norm-referenced, it seems important for music therapists to consider the need for more norm-referenced music therapy assessments.

The MATADOC (Magee et al., 2014) has been compared to a standardized reference measure, the Sensory Modality Assessment and Rehabilitation Technique (SMART). SMART has been validated in comparison to physician diagnosis and the Western Neuro Sensory Stimulation Profile (Gill-Thwaites & Munday, 2004). This research demonstrating the validity of MATADOC to assess response levels from persons with disorders of consciousness is a milestone in music therapy assessment development, the first standardized music therapy assessment measurement tool.

Assessment for Various Populations
Children with Special Needs

Carpente's IMCAP-ND assessment (2013), based on the Developmental, Individual-Difference, Relationship (DIR)/Floortime model of Greenspan (1992), offers another innovative approach to work with children. The Individualized Music Therapy Assessment Profile, or IMTAP (Baxter et al., 2007), was developed to assess strengths and needs of children and adolescents with special needs and is used in schools and by many music therapists working in private practice.

The Special Education Music Therapy Assessment Process (SEMTAP, Brunk & Coleman, 2000; Coleman & Brunk, 2003) was developed in response to the need of music therapists working in public school settings to be able to determine whether music therapy is *required* in order for a student to benefit from their academic placement. The authors indicate that the SEMTAP is a standardized process rather than a standardized assessment tool and that this distinction is important in that it allows each therapist to effectively communicate their findings to the child's parents and service providers in a consistent manner. In the SEMTAP, the emphasis is on testing a student's response to certain tasks that are specifically connected to already-existing objectives in the IEP. An assessment report from an assessment process following the SEMTAP model is shown in Table 5.3. This report has been adapted from an actual report using the SEMTAP model. All identifying features have been changed for confidentiality.

To summarize, this assessment has the following features:

- Focus: prescriptive;
- Domains: somatic, behavioral, skill, affective, interactional;

- Sources of musical information: improvising, performing or re-creating, composing, listening;
- Method of data collection and analysis: descriptive written summary;
- Reporting findings: written report; see Table 5.3 for an example.

Table 5.3
Assessment Report Using SEMTAP Approach

Student Name: Judy
DOB: Mar. 22, 2008
Grade: Kindergarten
Address:
School:
District:
Dates of Assessment: Aug. 10 and Aug. 14, 2014
Evaluator: Barbara L. Wheeler, PhD, MT-BC

Purpose of Assessment
To determine if music therapy, as a related service, provides significant assistance or motivation for the student to perform IEP skills.

Elements of Assessment
Review of most recent IEP
Interviews with IEP team members and supportive staff
Observation in two nonmusical settings
Preparation of a music therapy assessment session
Administration of a music therapy assessment session
Preparation of a written report

Classroom Observation
Judy was observed in two settings. The first, on Aug. 10, was in an outdoor art lesson where the children were "water painting." Judy worked alone and was quite focused on the project. She often sang to herself while painting. She did not interact with or appear to notice the other children. She did not indicate, either verbally or with eye contact, recognition of the teachers or respond to a greeting. She was also observed on Aug. 14 in a physical education class. This was held on the outside playground. At the beginning of the observation, she had been asked to leave the swing and come to where the class was listening to the teacher give instructions. She was resistive to this, but when her regular classroom aide assisted her, she came willingly. As soon as the children were allowed to go to various playground activities, she went back to the swing and remained there for the duration of the class. She used the swing appropriately, several times trying new ways to get it to move (such as twisting). She did not interact with or show any awareness of others, children or staff.

Review of IEP and IEP Goals
Judy's IEP indicated that, in the communication area, she speaks often but does not use speech appropriately to request items. Cognitively, she has problems with basic pre-academic skills such as identifying shapes, colors, and letters. Socially, she seldom makes eye contact and generally participates only individually in activities without exhibiting cooperative behavior. Physical and behavioral skills were felt to be progressing well and thus were not prioritized to be addressed in the music therapy assessment.

Music Therapy Assessment Results
Communication Skills
IEP goal assessed: Judy will demonstrate effective communication skills in the area of requesting preferred items.

Judy verbalized "Hello, Judy" very clearly and appropriately in response to an improvised hello song. Her response was supported by the structure of the song, which included the words, the request that she repeat them, and a space for her response. She did not consistently verbalize requests (for instruments or songs) as asked, nor did she verbally label objects so that her words could be understood.

Cognitive Skills
IEP goal assessed: Judy will demonstrate effective object naming in the areas of shape naming.

Judy was asked to point to shapes, letters, and colors. While she pointed willingly, she was not always correct in her choices, particularly for shapes. The structure of songs (rhythm, melody, and spaces) appeared to help her structure some of her responses, even when they were not correct.

Social Skills
IEP goal assessed: Judy will demonstrate effective social skills in the area of making eye contact.

Judy often does not make eye contact when speaking or when spoken to. On several occasions, she made eye contact as part of singing or another musical interaction.

Results
Judy demonstrates positive responses in the following skill areas in response to music stimuli:
Verbalizations
Identifying colors, shapes, letters
Eye contact

Recommendations
Judy responds well to various musical stimuli, including singing, playing instruments, and movement to music. She verbalized "Hello, Judy" very clearly and appropriately during a hello song. The structure of songs seemed to help her structure cognitive responses (recognition of colors, shapes, letters), even when they were incorrect. Eye contact occurred as part of singing and in other musical interactions. She appears motivated and structured by musical activities. Thus, music therapy is a viable means of working toward her educational needs, and it is recommended that weekly music therapy services be included in her IEP.

Suggested Goals and Objectives

Goal 1: Judy will demonstrate effective communication skills in the area of requesting preferred items.

Objective 1a: When given a prompt, Judy will verbalize two requests for instruments during the music therapy session for 3 consecutive probes.

Objective 1b: Judy will independently verbalize two requests for instruments during the music therapy session for 3 consecutive probes.

Goal 2: Judy will demonstrate effective object naming in the areas of shape naming.

Objective 2a: When presented with the following shapes—circle, square, triangle, rectangle, star, heart, diamond—Judy will correctly choose named shapes for 3 consecutive probes.

Objective 2b: When presented with a shape, Judy will say the name of the shape for 3 consecutive trials per shape.

Goal 3:   Judy will demonstrate effective social skills in the area of making eye contact.
Objective 3a: When given a prompt to "look at me," Judy will hold eye contact for 3 or more seconds for 3 consecutive probes.
Objective 3b: Judy will hold eye contact for 3 or more seconds when instruction begins with no verbal prompt for 3 consecutive probes.

Assessment report submitted by:
Barbara L. Wheeler, PhD, MT-BC

Layman, Hussey, and Laing (2002) designed the Beech Brook Music Therapy Assessment for Severely Emotionally Disturbed Children. This assessment measures four domains: (a) behavioral/social functioning (including play skills, attention to task, attempting activities, impulse control, compliance with structure, eye contact, and personal boundaries), (b) emotional responsiveness (including facial affect, coping skills, handling mistakes, and display of affection), (c) language/communication abilities (including response to simple directions, self-expression, expressive language, response to praise, and answering questions), and (d) music skills (musical awareness, responses to music, responses to cue, imitation, and vocal inflection). The authors measured responses along a continuum that ranged from defensiveness/withdrawn to disruptive/intrusive, with target behaviors assuming the middle range of the continuum. Examples from their scale, one for behavioral/social and another for musical, are shown in Table 5.4. The authors indicated that their assessment tool fared well in a pilot application, with good reliability (Layman, Hussey, & Laing, 2002). They stressed the importance of using language in the assessment process and resulting documentation that is easily understood by clinicians other than music therapists, in addition to pursuing development and use of a standardized assessment approach in order to advance research.

To summarize, this assessment has the following features:

- Focus: descriptive, prescriptive;
- Domains: behavioral, skill, affective, interactional;
- Sources of musical information: improvising, performing or re-creating, listening;
- Method of data collection and analysis: rating scales;
- Reporting findings: written summary, with results communicated to child's treatment team.

Table 5.4
Beech Brook Music Therapy Assessment for Severely Emotionally Disturbed Children, Sample Areas Assessed (Layman, Hussey, & Laing, 2002)
Used with permission from the American Music Therapy Association.

Behavioral/Social

Play Skills

Defensive/Withdrawn		**Target Behavior**	**Disruptive/Intrusive**	
2	1	0	1	2
Did not participate or play instruments; appeared afraid, tired, shy	Demonstrated some interaction (parallel play)	Consistently took turns with therapist (cooperative play)	Insisted on own turn/way 1–2 times in session; did not take turns with therapist 1–2 times	Frequently insisted on own turn/way throughout session (overpowering); did not take turns

Musical

Musical Awareness

2	1	0	1	2
Inconsistently altered tempo and/or dynamic to match outside stimulus when given 1 prompt or cue	Consistently altered tempo and/or dynamic to match outside stimulus when given 1 prompt or cue	Consistently altered tempo and/or dynamic to match outside stimulus independently	Did not alter tempo and/or dynamic to match outside stimulus, even when given prompts/cues	Displayed overpowering, loud dynamics throughout session

Defensive/Withdrawn   **Target Behavior**   **Disruptive/Intrusive**

Building on their experiences with the Beech Brook assessment described above and used with individual children, Layman, Hussey, and Reed (2013) developed a group treatment assessment focusing on communication, emotion, behavior, and social skills.

Adolescents and Adults with Developmental Disabilities

Polen (1985) developed an assessment for adults with developmental disabilities, the Music Therapy Assessment for Adults with Developmental Disabilities, a summary of which is shown in Table 5.5. In this assessment, the therapist observes and documents musical responses of the client and interprets them to determine musical and nonmusical strengths, needs, and interests. This information is then used in planning the client's treatment. Rather than include the complete checklist, descriptive information is provided on the domains tested under a broad range of headings: sensorimotor, cognitive, communication, and affective/emotional development.

To summarize, this assessment has the following features:

- Focus: descriptive, prescriptive;
- Domains: somatic, behavioral, affective, interactional;
- Sources of musical information: improvising, performing or re-creating;
- Method of data collection and analysis: checklist;
- Reporting findings: written report submitted to client chart; verbal report presented to team at treatment planning meeting.

Table 5.5
Music Therapy Assessment for Adults with Developmental Disabilities (Polen, 1985)
Used with permission.

Sensorimotor Development
In this portion of the assessment, areas that are addressed include:

- Gross motor: positioning (of client or instruments), hand dominance, ability to maintain a steady beat at varying tempos (hands separately, hands together, hands alternating), ability to cross midline;
- Fine motor: functional grasp (varying diameter), digital control (finger isolation, single-finger and alternating finger patterns on piano, plucking guitar strings);
- Diaphragmatic motor: lip closure, produces tones vocally or on a horn, ability to sustain tones vocally or instrumentally.

Cognitive Development
This section of the assessment addresses a broad range of skills, from basic concepts to more sophisticated areas of academic knowledge and classification skills. It is often the case that much of this section may not be presented to a client based on their functioning level.

- Attending skills: can sustain active involvement in tasks (instrumental, vocal, movement, verbal), ability to indicate preferences through sustained engagement;
- Recognition skills: recognizes familiar people or objects (verbally/nonverbally), remembers name or function of new instrument from start to end of session and from session to session;
- Recall skills: can imitate simple rhythm patterns on like-timbred (drum/drum) and unlike-timbred (piano/drum) instruments, ability to imitate complex (longer or syncopated) rhythm patterns on like-timbred (drum/drum) and unlike-timbred (piano/drum) instruments, recalls function of hello and good-bye songs;
- Choice-making: can choose between two, among three, open-ended, self-initiated;
- Basic academics: abilities in areas such as reading, writing, colors, numbers, temporal relationships, spatial relationships.

Communication Development

Areas addressed in this section include not only receptive and expressive communication skills but also preverbal and nonverbal communication, areas in which music therapy may be able to offer information regarding the client that other disciplines may not be able to access as readily.

- Receptive communication: ability to follow simple (one-step) and complex (multistep) directives given verbally or musically;
- Expressive communication: modes of communication used (verbal, gestures, sign, communication device, etc.); sings "hello," "good-bye," name, and so on; creates lyrics to a song in phrases or sentences;
- Preverbal/nonverbal communication: imitation skills (nonsense syllables, speech rhythms [by beating them on a drum or by vocally sounding the number of beats]), ability to vocalize responsively in tonality, ability to vocalize a sequence of pitches responsively, ability to vocalize in phrases performing auditory closure.

Affective/Emotional Development

This section of the assessment draws much of its information from engaging the client in improvisation experiences. Many of the comments that may appear in this section of a formal report might also seem appropriate for the Communication area, as the two domains share common ground in improvisation experiences.

- Verbal expression of emotion: identifies various emotions (anger, sadness, happiness, etc.) in music, identifies various emotions in relation to self (verbally or musically), as well as causations;
- Nonverbal expression of emotion through musical creativity: initiates original rhythmic or melodic patterns; initiates changes in tempo, dynamics, or meter; explores use of instruments; improvises instrumentally, vocally, or through movement; initiates musical jokes or games.

Snow (2009) developed an assessment and piloted it with eight adults, ages 20–40, with developmental disabilities. This pilot study demonstrated higher scores for clients with higher intellectual functioning, suggesting it is useful with this group.

Adults with Psychiatric Disorders

Several music therapy assessments have been developed for adults with psychiatric disorders. Braswell, Brooks, DeCuir, Humphrey, Jacobs, and Sutton (1983, 1986) used the Music/Activity Therapy Intake Assessment for Psychiatric Patients to examine the attitudes of clients with psychiatric problems, examining self-concept, interpersonal relationships, and altruism/optimism. Cohen and Gericke (1972) devised an assessment that combined clinical observation with information on musical ability, leading to recommendations about treatment.

Cassity and Cassity (2006) surveyed clinical training directors for information on areas of nonmusic behavior that they assessed and treated most frequently during music therapy sessions. They then asked them to write two patient problems assessed and treated most often for each area and two music therapy interventions used for each of these problems. They developed and organized this into a comprehensive manual, *Multimodal Psychiatric Music Therapy for Adults, Adolescents, and Children: A Clinical Manual*, 3rd edition.

In an assessment focusing on music experiences and responses, Pavlicevic and Trevarthen (1989) analyzed joint musical improvisations of clients with schizophrenia and depression. They were interested in whether there were differences in levels of musical contact of adults with differing psychiatric diagnoses. Baker, Silverman, and MacDonald (2016) developed a scale for assessing the meaningfulness of the songwriting experience to clients. This scale functions as an evaluative assessment, as it measures the outcome of an intervention and could be used to compare responses from one session to the next.

Older Adults with Age-Related Needs

Hintz (2000) describes a music therapy assessment that addresses client strengths, needs, and functioning levels and can be utilized in both long-term care and rehabilitation settings. The tool specifically targets the following areas in the skill domain: expressive musical skills, receptive musical skills, behavioral/psychosocial skills, motor skills, and cognitive/memory skills. Results of the testing are then interpreted and used in determining placement in music therapy services and specific treatment and program recommendations.

The Musical Assessment of Gerontologic Needs and Treatment: The MAGNET Survey (Adler, 2001) was designed to correlate with the Minimum Data Set (MDS), a multidisciplinary assessment used for treatment planning in long-term care facilities. Background information, musical preferences, and observable behaviors are collected in the initial part of the survey. The following areas are assessed in the session and included on the assessment form: cognition; emotional status; memory; motor skills; musical participation; musical preferences; musical skills; observable behaviors; reality orientation; sensory processing, planning, and task execution; singing; social interactions; and speech and communication. The assessment leads to a treatment plan, also included on the assessment form. It includes a model session from which the information needed to complete the assessment can be gained. This assessment is useful for in-depth assessment when time allows.

Norman (2012) has developed a more concise assessment for use with older adults in nursing care which complements the MDS process and can be done in an individual or group music therapy session. Keough, King, and Lemmerman (2016) used a demonstration project to develop a small group approach to assessment of persons with Alzheimer's disease that has been used as an evaluative assessment to measure change.

People in Medical Settings

Approaches that have been taken to assessment in medical settings include biographical interview (Dileo & Bradt, 1999; Zabin, 2005), rating scales (Loewy, 1999; Loewy, MacGregor, Richards, & Rodriguez, 1997), interpretation of musical materials (Dileo & Bradt, 1999; Loewy, 1999), and standardized physiological and psychological measures (Lane, 1991; Sandrock & James, 1989).

Scalenghe and Murphy's (2000) music therapy assessment in the managed care environment provides a comprehensive descriptive assessment of clients, divided into nine major areas previously outlined in this chapter (history of present illness, behavioral observations, motor skills, communication skills, cognitive skills, auditory perceptual skills, social skills, specific musical behaviors, and summary and recommendations). The purpose of this assessment is twofold: (a) to describe the skills of the client in these areas and consequently identify therapeutic goals, and (b) to meet the assessment requirements of the managed care setting and, in so doing, advocate for the inclusion of music therapy in the therapeutic milieu.

Zabin (2005), Dileo and Bradt (1999), and Loewy (1999) describe qualitative, semistructured interview approaches to assessing clients. Zabin, in work with hospice patients who were near death, describes how she begins each assessment with a brief interview (with the patient, patient's family, or both) in order to understand the patient's background, musical interests, and present situation. Based upon this interview, Zabin immediately begins singing or playing music for the patient and his or her family (if they are present), and additional assessment information is gathered inductively as the session unfolds. In their work with children experiencing severe pain, Dileo and Bradt (1999) describe the collection of medical, psychosocial, and musical information from traditional sources. However, an additional emphasis is on understanding how the patient uses musical media to express his or her experience of the pain, "the meaning of the pain, nonverbal characteristics of the pain, as well as evidence of pain-related suffering (i.e., feelings of helplessness, hopelessness, etc.)" (p. 184). Based upon this information, music therapy goals and treatment are designed to address the child's pain experience.

The purpose of Loewy's (1999) music therapy pain assessment is to "understand and feel the pain of the patient as well as it can be defined by him or her" (p. 195). In addition to asking patients to comprehensively describe their pain, she also has them improvise their pain because these improvisations "provide clues on how to address physical aspects of the tension" (p. 195). By playing with her patients, Loewy is also able to assess the types of interventions needed to ameliorate the patient's pain and the therapist's role in doing so.

The Computer-Based Music Perception Assessment for Children (CMPAC) and Music Attentiveness Screening Assessment (MASA) (Wolfe & Waldon, 2009), described earlier in the chapter, can be used to gather "initial information on children admitted to pediatric services [and] assist the therapist in making appropriate music therapy referral decisions and preparing music therapy interventions that will be effective for particular children undergoing specific kinds of medical procedures" (p. 11). The authors suggest that the use of computer technology in these assessments is desirable, since time is of the essence in acute hospitalization. They also describe two nonmusic tools that can assist in assessing and monitoring a child during music therapy interventions. The first of these is the Observation Scale of Behavioral Distress (OSBD), consisting of eight categories of behavioral distress that were developed to observe children undergoing invasive procedures such as bone marrow aspirations and lumbar punctures (Jay, Ozolins, Elliott, & Caldwell, 1983, as cited in Wolfe & Waldon, 2009). The second nonmusic tool that they describe is the Simple Computer Recording Interface for Behavioral Evaluation (SCRIBE), which records the frequency and duration of observed events (Duke & Stammen, 2006, as cited in Wolfe & Waldon, 2009). All of these computer-based tools are used in pediatric music therapy as well as other areas.

Thompson, Arnold, and Murray (1990) describe a systematic, hierarchical assessment for patients who have recently suffered a cerebrovascular accident (CVA) to determine their current level of functioning. Typically taking three 30-minute sessions to complete, this descriptive assessment covers six major areas of functioning: (a) orientation (self-recognition and memory), (b) visual (memory, perception, discrimination), (c) auditory (identification of sounds, discrimination of sounds, abstract thinking related to songs, counting, and spelling), (d) motor (identification of body parts, sensory awareness, body integration, body use—musical and nonmusical), (e) communication (presence of various communication disorders such as aphasia and agnosia; articulation; respiration; phonation; vocal range), and (f) social (affect, range of social behaviors, self-control, self-concept).

Jeong and Lesiuk (2011) used melodic contour as a basis for the Music-Based Attention Assessment (MAA), created for use with patients after traumatic brain injury (TBI). Further testing resulted in the development of the MAA-R, a valid and reliable 45-item assessment of auditory attention (Jeong, 2013). *Medical Music Therapy for Pediatrics in Hospital Settings* (2008) and *Medical Music Therapy for Adults in Hospital Settings* (2010), both edited by Hanson-Abromeit and Colwell, include many examples of assessment for different medical diagnoses.

Although not specifically developed by music therapists, assessments of music-related medical conditions have also been developed. These include the diagnostic assessment of amusia (Berman, 1981), musicogenic epilepsy (Critchley, 1977), and music alexia (Horikoshi et al., 1997).

Summary

Music therapy assessment is a process that involves observing the client making or listening to music under specific musical conditions that enable the therapist to assess the client's abilities. It has one or more of the following goals: diagnosis, prescription, interpretation, description, or evaluation (Bruscia, 1993, 2003). It involves focusing on one or more of the following domain areas: biographical, somatic, behavioral, skill, affective, or interactional (Bruscia, 1993).

Assessment information is gathered from one or more of the following four musical sources: improvising, performing or re-creating, composing, listening.

The assessment process usually involves the following procedural steps: (a) receiving a referral, (b) gathering background information, (c) determining the goals and type of assessment, (d) implementing the assessment, (e) interpreting the data, and (f) creating a report and communicating the findings.

Once the assessment is completed, the therapist can make a number of decisions about how to proceed with the client. These include addressing the following:

- Is the client suitable for music therapy?
- Should the client be seen individually or in a group?
- What are the goals of music therapy treatment?
- What kinds of musical experiences should the client be undertaking (e.g., listening, improvising)?

Although it is easy to think of assessment as a distinct phase of the therapeutic process, in actuality, assessment is usually an ongoing part of the treatment process—while you gather an understanding of the client before you begin treatment, you are constantly reassessing the client according to their responses in sessions, and in this way you are expanding upon and clarifying your original understanding of the client.

Assignments—Client Assessment

These assignments should help you to better understand assessment and develop your skills:

- Use the General Behavior Checklist (see Table 5.1) to observe the behavior of one of the clients in a session. Write down what you find, then summarize what you have discovered that could be useful in determining the treatment needs of the client.
- Select a client from the session that you are observing. Select two domains (biographical, somatic, behavioral, skill, personality or sense of self, affective, or interactional) in which you feel that it would be useful to have information. Determine the sources of musical information—improvising, performing or re-creating, composing, listening—that would be useful for gathering the desired information. Then specify one way that you could use each of the relevant sources

of musical information to gather information that you would desire. Write down what you would do; at this point, you will not actually perform any aspect of the assessment.

- Select one client from your clinical setting. Then select an existing assessment that could be relevant for this person; it can be one that was described or mentioned in the chapter or one that is already used in your clinical setting. Select one or two domain areas and identify the sources of musical information in which the client would need to be engaged in order to gather the data. (This will be easier to do with some populations than others, as assessments are more plentiful in some areas than others and the information to be assessed is also more accessible to a student in the process of learning how to do this.)
- Find three music therapy assessments in the literature. You may use assessments that were referred to in this chapter, except for those that were described in detail. Examine the ways in which they have been constructed. Identify the purpose, domains, and sources of musical information. Then discuss the relevance to your clients of these existing assessments to your clients.
- Carry out a prescriptive or descriptive assessment in your clinical setting. Assess one client in two or three domains. Discuss the results of your assessment and their implications for planning the treatment needs of the clients with your clinical supervisor. Are they in agreement with your findings? What do you learn about improving your implementation and interpretation skills as a result of this consultation, and how does it inform your efforts with the following assignment?
- Reflect on your experiences with assessment up to this point. Write about the areas in which you feel that your assessment concepts and procedures have been successful in gaining information that you need. Then write about areas in which you feel that your assessments have been less successful. Analyze these as to whether there are problems in how you conceptualize the assessment areas or how you carry them out. Develop a plan for making them work more successfully. (This process of self-assessment is the same that you will be encouraged to follow in other aspects of your music therapy clinical work.)

Acknowledgment

Anthony Meadows was the primary author of this chapter in the first edition of this book. The current chapter is based on that chapter, and we acknowledge his work and thank him for his expertise and insights into music therapy assessment.

6 Goals and Objectives

Completing an assessment provides information about the client's needs, strengths, and interests. From this information, the music therapist formulates a treatment plan that is relevant and meaningful to the client. The first part of a treatment plan is to determine the long-range intent or purpose of the treatment. The next step is the establishment of goals with accompanying objectives for treatment. Objectives are rooted in the musical experiences used in the session.

Not all music therapists work in this concrete manner; some music therapists approach treatment with an open-ended intent but without specified measurable goals and objectives. This more open approach is not common in healthcare institutions or schools, where measurable outcomes are often needed to meet administrative and reimbursement goals. Whether a music therapist operates within a framework that uses concrete goals and objectives or works to help the client evolve through the musical interaction without having predetermined goals and objectives in mind, it is essential that the music therapy have a focus or intent. This focus often forms the basis for the goals for music therapy.

Establishing Goals

Music therapy goals may be established in several ways. One is to base them on the findings of the assessment. In some settings, the treatment team establishes goals for the client. In these cases, the music therapist does not do a formal assessment but formulates goals for music therapy based on the team's assessment and goals, together with a less formal assessment gleaned from the first contacts with the client as well as what is found in the client records.

The task of writing goals has been developed not only by healthcare professionals but also by business managers. The SMART (specific, measurable, attainable, realistic, and time-based) mnemonic grew out of the MBO (management by objective) process and was originally associated with business guru Peter Drucker (Bogue, 2005). SMART was first published in a management journal by Doran in 1981. Wade (2009) suggests that goal-setting is a complex process but that SMART and SMARTER (ethical and recorded) can be helpful in designing goals that are meaningful and relevant for persons receiving rehabilitative care. (Note that the letters in SMART and SMARTER have been assigned various words over the years but the intent remains constant: to help goal writers clarify the language of a goal.)

The American Music Therapy Association *Standards of Clinical Practice* defines a goal quite broadly as "a projected outcome of a treatment plan" while defining an objective as "one of a series of progressive accomplishments leading toward goal attainment" (2013b, n.p.). Thus, in music therapy, a goal may be a long-range outcome (or purpose statement) or it may be a goal for a specified period of time. If the work is being done in a school setting, the goal may be for the academic year. The music therapist might set short-term goals (sometimes referred to as "benchmarks") leading to the accomplishment of that overall goal but which are still stated in general terms, followed by specific objectives as steps toward the achievement of the goal(s).

An effectively written goal statement includes a level of specificity about the direction in which change is sought, but without being too precise. It states the type of change that it is hoped that the client will make with enough precision that it establishes a focus and also communicates this to others who are concerned with the treatment process. The authors' preference is to be more specific than, for example, "improve socialization" or "develop communication," since such broad goals can elicit a myriad of responses. (The goal "improve socialization" could mean anything from an infant focusing a gaze on a caregiver to a young adult becoming more comfortable with interpersonal relationships appropriate in dating.) Therefore, such goals as "learn to take turns" or "decrease anxiety in a social situation" in the social realm and "increase frequency of eye contact" or "increase topic-based verbalizations" in the area of developing communication are more desirable.

Broad goals are useful in helping the therapist understand the area of treatment to be addressed. These might be thought of as *purpose statements* that help to define the overall intent of the therapy process. More specific goals help to define the desired outcome of the therapy. These goals provide a focus for the development of objectives that can be used to measure progress toward goals for each individual client.

Since goals may be stated somewhat differently in various settings, the music therapist will need to adapt the style of writing goals to what is appropriate in his or her setting. In some situations, therapists find it useful to have long-range as well as short-term goals. In this situation, the long-range goal may be for a year, with short-term goals for a period of several months or a semester. In some settings, these short-term goals may be for as little as 1 week or one session; thus, it becomes very important that these goals be stated clearly. These additional goal levels are not elaborated here but can be developed when the need arises using the principles discussed here. One of the best ways to learn how to write effective goals is to study the goal statements written by other music therapists and those in the particular treatment setting.

A useful goal conveys the direction of the desired change (e.g., improve, increase, decrease) and describes the targeted responses with a moderate degree of specificity. Goals will generally be appropriate for a period of time ranging from a single session to several months or more. In many treatment settings, goals have specific target dates based on the pattern of treatment plan review for that setting. For example, students in school have Individualized Education Plans (IEPs) that are reviewed annually, while residents of long-term care facilities have care plans that are reviewed quarterly. Therefore, goals for practicum work may continue for the entire semester or be altered according to the pattern of the treatment setting.

Some sample goals include:

- Improve visual tracking,
- Develop one-word response,
- Follow two-step command,
- Increase reality orientation,
- Increase verbal interaction,
- Improve range of motion,
- Increase creative self-expression,
- Increase independent use of leisure time,
- Increase appropriate verbal responses,
- Increase verbalization of thoughts and feelings regarding the current medical situation.

Still another perspective is that of music-centered music therapy and the premise that establishing purely musical goals is clinically valid. Certainly changes in musical response (such as the ability to synchronize with the basic beat, to follow changes in music, to recall and imitate melodic lines, and so on) are easy enough to observe and document. The historical foundations of this way of thinking can be found in the works of music therapy pioneers Helen Bonny, Paul Nordoff, and Clive Robbins. Some current resources that we recommend if you are interested in reading and learning more about this include two books by Aigen, *Music-Centered Music Therapy* (2005b) and *The Study of Music Therapy: Current Issues and Concepts* (2014b), and the articles "Music-Centered Dimensions of Nordoff-Robbins Music Therapy" by Aigen (2014a) and "Individual Music-Centered Assessment Profile for Neurodevelopmental Disorders (IMCAP-ND): New Developments in Music-Centered Evaluation" by Carpente (2014).

Establishing Objectives

Once goals have been established, the music therapist usually identifies objectives. These objectives define outcomes expected to occur in the session and will indicate whether or not the goal is being achieved. Objectives are thus small, observable, and measurable. Since objectives are responses that you expect to observe in the session, they will be specific to the musical strategies that you plan to employ and will change from session to session as your procedures change. A way of thinking about formulating objectives requires an analysis of the musical experiences planned for a session. How do the elements of the music address the goals? What responses will the client(s) display to demonstrate that they are moving toward the achievement of the goals? Goodman (2007) suggests that the music therapist needs to have a grasp of the goals and objectives and how they are embedded into the musical experiences of the session in order to respond spontaneously in the session while remaining focused on the goals and objectives. Berger (2009) also argues for this perspective: "Goals and objectives developed from [a] comprehensive (scientific and clinical), in-depth understanding of causes and deficits from both the physiological and music treatment perspectives help target the work specifically as *treatment* with music" (Defining Goals and Objectives, paragraph 1).

In addition, objectives will often change from session to session as the client accomplishes each objective and comes closer to reaching the goals. Unlike objectives, goals are unlikely to change quickly.

One format for establishing objectives consists of three parts: (a) conditions, (b) behavior, and (c) criteria. As can be seen in the samples below, the *conditions* refer to what is expected to occur in the session that will provide the opportunity for the behavior to be observed, the *behavior* is what is targeted for the client to do at that time, and the *criteria* indicate how well or how many times the behavior is expected to be performed.

Sample objectives, defined under the previously listed goals that they support, include:

Goal: Improve visual tracking
Objectives:
1) When instrument is moved horizontally in front of child's face, child will follow instrument with eyes 80% of the time.
2) When instrument is moved vertically in front of child, child will follow with gaze 2 out of 3 times.

Goal: Increase verbal interaction
    Objectives:
    1) During planned break in lyrics of song, client will face another client and answer the question posed by the song with a maximum of one prompt.
    2) When requested by therapist, client will verbally state how she feels.

Goal: Increase independent use of leisure time
    Objectives:
    1) When offered a list of resources available, the client will choose one musical activity for use during leisure time.
    2) When provided with a preferred musical resource, the client will report use of the resource between sessions, along with a log to document use.

As mentioned above, the objectives are expected to change over time. Keeping in mind that many clients (as well as nonclients) do not change quickly, the changes may be slow and gradual. In short-term settings where contact with the client is brief, the objectives need to be constructed to allow the therapist to identify a small change that can be defined as a step toward the desired goal. While some objectives will typically change over time (an objective may change from "when therapist plays an instrument, child will turn in the direction of the sound 30% of the time" to "when therapist plays an instrument, child will reach for the instrument 30% of the time), in other cases only the percentage of desired responses will change to reflect an improvement (the objective may change from "when therapist plays an instrument, child will turn in the direction of the sound 30% of the time" to "when therapist plays an instrument, child will turn in the direction of the sound 60% of the time"). In the case of people with progressive illnesses such as dementia, the objectives may not yield changes in a positive direction; indeed, the client may lose ground in a number of areas. The goal of the music therapy in this latter case might be to preserve functioning for as long as possible.

Part of the value of having objectives is that they help the music therapist focus on how much of the behavior should be sought or how well the client is expected to do at any particular time. Properly set objectives will be achievable over a period of time. If the client is consistently not meeting the objectives that have been set, it is likely that the objectives were not set correctly. In these cases, the therapist should reevaluate the expectations and set new objectives.

Once the objectives are properly stated, they are not difficult to measure. It is through measuring objectives that we determine when to change them and also whether the goals are being met. It is important for goals and objectives to be reviewed regularly and changed as the client's responses warrant.

The following illustrations provide a detailed example of two different formats for writing goals and objectives. For another example, see Ritter-Cantesanu (2014) for a comprehensive example of her goals and objectives from an IEP in a special education setting. The first example below describes a purpose statement and long- and short-term goals that might be found in a long-term care setting (nursing care facility), and the second offers specific goals and objectives written for a music therapy session with preschool children. Note that the objectives written for a session are much more specific than those written for the overall treatment plan in long-term care. Both, however, meet the SMART criteria.

Long-Term Care Treatment Plan Goals and Objectives

The overall purpose of music therapy treatment for this group of residents in long-term care is to improve the quality of life for those living within the community. Long-range goals can be established that are more specific than the overall purpose, defining what a better quality of life in long-term care means. These long-range goals would be broken down into short-term goals that are more specific, measurable outcomes. These are the goal-oriented statements that best match the SMART style of goal-setting. The therapist might then also create specific objectives for the music therapy session that could yield weekly data after each session.

Richard is newly admitted to a long-term care community and has been isolating himself in his room. The staff referred him to music therapy because the only thing that brings him out of his room is musical entertainment. After assessing Richard's strengths and needs, you decide to invite him to your weekly self-expression group. The group consists of 10–12 residents who are invited to sing, play instruments, and do songwriting and improvisation together as a platform for sharing themselves with one another and building relationships.

You establish the following goals for Richard:

Purpose of treatment
  1) Decrease stress of living in long-term care community.

Long-range goals (related goals that are time-specific)
  1) Increase participation in scheduled events by (date could be 3–6 months away).
  2) Build social relationship with peer(s) by (date could be 3–6 months away or longer, depending upon the music therapist's knowledge of the environment),
  3) Increase self-expression through arts programming by (date could be 3–6 months away).

Short-term goals would be the more specific, measurable outcomes. For example ...
  1) Increase participation in scheduled events by (date).
     a. Richard will attend a minimum of one music-related program per week by (date).
        i. Richard will participate in weekly music therapy session(s) by actively engaging in one experience (singing, playing, creating, moving to music).
  2) Build social relationship with peer(s) by (date).
     a. Richard will build a social relationship with at least one peer by (date). (This might a good place to think about how you will know if this has occurred. In some settings, the phrase "as evidenced by" [AEB] is used to delineate the specific observable behaviors that will be the indication that the goal has been met.) In this case: Richard will build ... AEB self-report that he enjoys doing activities with Mr. X or by his desire to sit with specific residents at events.
        i. Richard will interact with peers in weekly music therapy group by sharing a memory or offering an idea for a group song.
  3) Increase self-expression through arts programming by (date).
     a. Richard will participate in a choir or small singing group with peers by (date).
        i. Richard will use songs or instruments to express himself in weekly music therapy sessions.

In this case, the music therapist is working toward specific nonmusical goals but has specific musical tasks for each weekly music therapy session that are leading toward those nonmusical goals. These tasks include those listed above as the basis of the group: singing, playing, improvising, and songwriting.

Session-Specific Goals and Objectives for a Preschool Group

Goal: To develop expressive language
Objectives:
1) Child will sing at least six phrases (two words or more) along with the MT, using intelligible speech during the session.
2) Child will speak at least four phrases (two words or more), using intelligible speech during the session with cues from the MT.

Goal: To increase self-control
Objectives:
1) Child will play the drum softly for one verse of the song sung by the MT.
2) Child will clap only twice at phrase ends in "Let's make music now," with modeling by the MT.
3) Child will clap up to three out of the six claps during "The Very Hungry Caterpillar," as cued by the MT.

Goal: To increase attention
Objectives:
1) Child will sing along with the MT during four out of the eight interventions.
2) Child will verbally respond to at least three questions asked by the MT during "The Very Hungry Caterpillar" and "Wheels on the Bus."
3) Child will follow directions given by the MT during 100% of interventions.

Different Formats for Different Settings

It is of crucial importance to develop your abilities to establish appropriate and meaningful music therapy goals and objectives, to create effective methods for implementing goals, and to design workable strategies for obtaining data and documenting your work. Once you have developed these skills, you may find yourself delivering services in settings that have very different requirements and needs related to the development, implementation, and ongoing documentation and evaluation of clinical intervention.

One example of this is the recent increase of music therapists working in settings where service providers focus on determining the desires and interests of clients. While the goals *(outcomes)* may ultimately be the same (e.g., to increase verbal interaction, improve range of motion), rather than establishing one goal and several objectives that may concentrate on what the client *will* do, the therapist may establish one plan or goal that encompasses several objectives *(skills)* that the client *wants* to do.

If the therapist is working in a setting where clients are able to actively participate in the development of their plans, this can be an exciting and interesting addition to the process of establishing a relationship and creating a truly meaningful method to help the person reach his or her goals. If, on the other hand, the therapist is working in a setting in which clients are unable to participate in this process due to cognitive, physical, communicative, and/or emotional challenges, the actual process of developing the plan may resemble that of developing the more traditional goals and objectives but will result in a different format.

Some examples of client-driven music therapy outcomes and skills are provided to help you familiarize yourself with the different formats. Always be aware that regardless of the format of documentation required by various agencies and regulations, as the person providing music therapy services, you need to have a focus in mind of how to implement the goals and document the responses of the client and the effectiveness of your strategies.

Music Therapy Outcome: Client wants to participate in music experiences that offer opportunities to engage in structured relaxation training, development of enhanced self-esteem, and further development of effective communication skills in social and learning experiences.

Skill-Building Areas for Documentation:

- Increase the length of time the client remains still (physically and verbally) during use of the Somatron® Wedge;
- Increase client's positive self-statements in response to questions from the therapist relating to client's effective use of the Somatron® in therapy, as well as relating to other experiences in therapy;
- Increase ability to engage in social and learning experiences with peers and adults immediately following therapy.

Music Therapy Outcome: Client wants to participate in music experiences that offer opportunities for further development of receptive and expressive communication skills, basic cognitive concepts, and enhanced self-expression.

Skill-Building Areas for Documentation:

- Learn and sing question/answer learning songs dealing with a variety of academic and social concepts;
- Increase independence in writing answers to question/answer learning songs;
- Increase the amount of time client sustains tones either vocally or through playing the single-reed horn;
- Increase frequency of participating in instrumental improvisations.

Music Therapy Outcome: Client wants to learn how to express herself more effectively and feel better about herself, as well as improve her ability to relax.

Skill-Building Areas for Documentation:

- Learn and sing new songs from the standard and popular repertoire, concentrating on breath support and articulation;
- Practice already-known question/answer learning songs as well as learn new ones dealing with a variety of academic and social concepts;
- Increase the amount of time during instrumental improvisations that client is actively using both hands functionally;
- Explore a wider variety of styles, rhythms, dynamics, and phrasing.

Assignments—Goals and Objectives

To develop your ability to write goals and objectives, consider the following:

- Look at the examples of goals and objectives presented in this chapter. What purpose or long-range goal might be the ultimate outcome of achieving a specific goal?
- Define a purpose statement for your current practicum population. Write at least three goals that address this purpose statement with accompanying objectives.

What kinds of musical experiences will help to move clients toward the achievement of these goals?

- If you are working with a group, state group goals and objectives as well as individual goals and objectives for two group members with differing needs. The goals for the group may be the same at times as those for individuals, but at other times they will be different but complementary. Discuss the two sets of goals with your supervisor or peers to help you think about how you might work on both group and individual goals in one session.

- If you are not yet setting goals and objectives, list three goals that you believe the therapist has established. Write them in the style suggested in this chapter. Then ask the therapist what his or her goals are. Compare your goals with those of the therapist, including things that you believe influenced discrepancies; do this in writing.

7 Planning and Implementing Music Therapy Strategies

One of the first questions that music therapy students usually have is: What do I *do* in a session? Although beginning students may not realize it, the real question is: What do I do *to meet the needs of the client?* And that question naturally leads to the question, *How* do I do what is required to meet the client's needs? This is the key question—it is what music therapy students work on and progress toward as they move through their music therapy education, and it is the focus of this chapter.

Much of the supervision that you will receive has to do with just this issue. As you plan a session, you will combine several music therapy strategies (also called *activities, experiences, interventions,* or *methods*) to form a session that allows you to work toward the goals and objectives that have been established. It is also important that each portion of the session be at an appropriate level for the client, be interesting and rewarding in order to encourage involvement, and help the client progress toward the goals and objectives.

The steps discussed in this chapter rely on the information gained from the assessment, as presented in Chapter 5, and then use the goals and objectives determined to be important, as discussed in Chapter 6, to develop music therapy sessions. In this chapter, you learn to plan the strategies or activities that you will use to work toward these goals and objectives. You will then take these strategies and formulate them into a session and discuss implementing and evaluating that session.

Music therapists use a variety of approaches to determine appropriate strategies for working with a client at the client's identified level of functioning. All are ways to help the client achieve his or her goals. All rely on information gained from the assessment and from ongoing observation.

We begin by looking at ways to determine appropriate strategies—what you need to accomplish through the strategy in light of the client's level of functioning—and how you sequence the steps in the activity itself. We will consider three different but related elements that may inform our decisions: (a) task analysis, (b) skill analysis, and (c) level of development. After looking at these, we will discuss criteria that can be used to evaluate whether the strategy is appropriate.

Two forms will assist you in planning strategies. The Strategy/Activity Form in Table 7.1 can be used to help to organize your planning. Although goals and objectives were discussed in Chapter 6 of this book, the definitions that Bruscia includes on this form may be useful and are quoted here:

Goal. A goal is a statement that describes the direction of the therapist's efforts and the end toward which that effort is directed. Grammatically, a goal consists of an infinitive phrase, a direct object, and the necessary modifiers (e.g., to eliminate self-injurious behaviors). Notice that the doer or implied agent is the therapist, not the client. The infinitive phrase reveals not only the current functioning level of the client, but also the direction of the therapist's efforts. For example, "to establish" implies that the client does not do something and that the therapist will work to elicit it for the first time; "to increase or decrease" implies that the client already does something and that the therapist will try to change the frequency of its occurrence; "to improve" implies that the client already does something but not very well and that the therapist will try to develop it further. The direct object and the modifiers give details about the areas of concern cited above.

Objective. An objective is a statement that describes what the client will be doing as a result of the therapist's efforts and as evidence that the goal has been achieved. Notice that the doer or agent here is the client rather than the therapist. Grammatically, an objective is a full sentence, starting with the phrase "The client will," followed by a verb that describes the client's actions, and modifying phrases which give details about the stimulus, reinforcement conditions, and desired frequency, accuracy, intensity, etc. Examples are: The client will sing back four-bar melodies with accurate pitch after one presentation, and, The client will play assigned instruments at the appropriate spot in the piece, without visual prompting. A goal has more than one objective when its accomplishment requires several steps or when the client needs to generalize the same objective from one situation or setting to another.

The Guidelines for Activity Planning in Table 7.2 will give you ideas to consider in planning for various populations. An additional resource that many have found useful for many aspects of planning and evaluating music therapy sessions, including student progress in conducting sessions, is *Music Techniques in Therapy, Counseling, and Special Education,* 3rd edition, by Standley and Jones (2007).

Table 7.1
Strategy/Activity Form (Bruscia, 1993)
Used with permission.

Date:
Music Title: The name of the song, instrumental piece, play, etc. Leave blank if there is no composition.
Source: Where you found the music or activity, including author, title, and page.
Population: The diagnostic classification of the clients for whom this activity was planned.
Activity Type or Title: Specify whether this is a greeting song, good-bye song, vocal call-and-response song, movement–action song, instrument action song, chant, song sung with instrumental accompaniment, instrumental ensemble, notated song or piece, structured movement to music, dance, etc.
Musical Characteristics: Describe the form of the song or piece; its rhythmic, melodic, and harmonic characteristics; how the parts are divided between the players; elaborateness of the score and accompaniment; difficulties that might be encountered by the client.
Skill Requirements: What skills will the client need to participate in this activity?
Areas of Concern: Each area of concern represents abilities and skills in a specific area of living. The most common are:
- *Sensorimotor development:* reflexive responses, sensory acuity or awareness (visual–motor, auditory–motor, fine motor, and gross motor skills).
- *Perceptual development:* auditory or visual perception of figure–ground, part–whole, same–different; identifying similarities (conserving) and differences (discriminating) between stimuli.
- *Cognitive development:* breadth, depth, and duration of attention; short- and long-term memory, learning style; academic concepts and skills; ability to make inferences or abstractions.
- *Behavior:* adaptive or maladaptive behaviors in a music setting; impulsivity,

destructiveness, aggression, etc.

- *Emotions:* range, variability, and appropriateness of feelings; expressivity; preferences, moods, etc.
- *Communication:* receptive and expressive abilities in speech, language, and other modalities.
- *Interpersonal:* awareness, sensitivity, intimacy, tolerance in relation to others; interactional skills; group skills; role behaviors; ability to form relationships.
- *Self-help:* toileting, dressing, eating, grooming, hygiene, clothing, safety.
- *Community living:* skills required for independent living, such as transportation, money management, shopping, etc.; appropriate use of leisure time; vocational pursuits, job skills, social behaviors at work, etc.
- *Medical:* abilities or skills necessitated by illness, medical treatment, or hospitalization.
- *Musical experience:* preferences; vocal or instrumental skills; practice habits; repertoire; ensemble skills; improvisational skills; musical tendencies when performing, improvising, or composing.
- *Creativity:* fluidity, divergence, originality, inventiveness.
- *Spiritual:* issues pertaining to religion, divine being, etc., that may be of concern to client.

Therapeutic Goals and Objectives
    Goal 1:
        Objectives:
    Goal 2:
        Objectives:
Environment: What instruments, props, furniture, materials, scores, cues, reinforcers, etc., will you and the client need for this activity? How will the room be arranged with regard to the equipment, furniture, open space, and people? What kind of atmosphere do you need?
Step-by-Step Method of Presentation: Describe in detail how you plan to engage the clients in this activity, including how you will break down the activity into steps; the verbal instructions you will give prior to each step; and the various prompts, cues, and supports you will give. Be very specific and complete about what you will say and what you will do as well as what you expect the clients to do at each step. Use this format:

    Step One:
        Therapist:
        Client:
    Step Two:
        Therapist:
        Client:
Activities That Precede and Follow:

Evaluation of Effectiveness of Strategy:

Table 7.2
Guidelines for Activity Planning (Bruscia, 1993)
Used with permission.

Every client population has its own problems and needs that will affect participation in music therapy. The following are some basic questions to ask when planning interventions.

Therapeutic Priorities: Identify the most important areas of concern, goals, and objectives when working with this population.

Medical Needs: Does the client have any medical conditions that contraindicate any form or level of participation in music therapy? What special precautions must be taken to ensure the medical safety of the client? Does the client have seizures? Is the client taking any medication, and, if so, what effects can be expected?

Physical Needs: What are the client's physical capabilities? Can he or she stand up; walk; sit up straight; use arms, hands, and fingers? Does the client have a visual or hearing impairment? Is he or she toilet-trained, able to indicate toileting needs, use toilet independently?

Environmental Needs: What special precautions should be taken in organizing the room or in the furniture and equipment in the room? How should clients and therapist be situated in space? What kind of physical atmosphere is needed?

Musical Needs: What kinds of musical experiences and activities are needed and preferred: listening, improvising, re-creative, creative? Should the media be vocal, instrumental, or movement? What styles of music are most appropriate and preferred? What kinds of musical direction and support are generally needed? Should the music be stimulative or sedative, flexible or structured?

Communication Needs: What kinds of instructions, cues, prompts, and communication supports do clients need? How will verbal and nonverbal forms of communication be used in tandem? How should instruction be paced and broken down? Is review necessary? What extra aids are needed?

Session Needs: Do clients need free-flowing or structured sessions? What kinds of warm-ups or preparations are needed before beginning? What are closure needs?

Emotional Needs: What kinds of emotional issues are likely to arise? How well do clients relate to therapist or others? What emotional needs must be met?

The basic and ongoing question is, How do I ensure the safety of the client while also addressing therapeutic needs?

Task Analysis

The assessment process will have helped you to gather information about the client and his or her level of functioning, interests, and so forth. It may be helpful to refer to Chapter 5, Client Assessment, to review some of this information. You then need to translate this information into appropriate strategies for working on the needs determined from the assessment. It is important that the strategies be sequenced correctly in order to help the client move from what he or she can do to what you are helping him or her learn to do. To accomplish this, you will often perform a task analysis. A task analysis is just what the name says: an analysis or breakdown of the task to be performed. It involves listing all of the steps that are involved in performing the task in the order in which they need to be accomplished. Webster (2016) gives concrete examples of task analyses for special education, and Watson and Wilson (2003) provide a comprehensive text that gives information on task analyses.

Task analyses can be conducted in various domains. Gagné and Briggs (1974) classify learned capabilities into intellectual skills, cognitive strategies, verbal information, attitudes, and motor skills. These domains are often used in the field of instructional design, from which task analyses have evolved.

Music therapists often do a task analysis in order to determine the sequence and the steps to follow to help the client reach a desired behavior. Presenting tasks in the proper sequence is important for any client or group of clients but is particularly important when working with people at lower levels of functioning, as these people are less able to catch on to or learn a skill that they have not been specifically taught. Therefore, in this section we will use an example of a task analysis with a lower-functioning client.

As a beginning music therapy student, you may become so focused on the goal (response, outcome) that you are attempting to elicit that you forget that there are actually many smaller steps that lead up to the desired response. By learning to look for these smaller steps, you will find that you are better able to organize experiences and present tasks in ways that provide for a more stimulating and successful session with the clients. Performing a task analysis is one fairly straightforward way to accomplish this.

As an example of the usefulness of a task analysis, think about a simple daily activity such as brushing your teeth. While the desired outcome is good oral hygiene as achieved through efficient brushing of teeth, a number of steps are required to reach that end result. Steps include:

- Gathering needed supplies (toothbrush, toothpaste, water, towel),
- Combining these supplies in the appropriate ways (squeezing toothpaste on toothbrush, applying toothbrush to teeth),
- The action needed to actually brush the teeth (grasping the toothbrush, the brushing motion, movement of the toothbrush to all areas of the mouth), and so on.

Miss one step—let's say letting the toothpaste fall into the sink rather than successfully squeezing it onto the bristles of the brush—and the end result, good oral hygiene, is not achieved.

Transfer this same skill set to the music therapy context. Suppose that you are working with a client for whom learning to brush his teeth is a goal. Perhaps he has achieved the skills needed for the earlier steps in the process but needs to develop enough hand coordination and strength to grasp the toothbrush and form the brushing motion. You have been asked to work on these skills in music therapy.

Since there are many things that can be done in music therapy to work on hand coordination and strength, we need to choose (at least) one strategy on which to focus. For our example, let's use playing the drum. Since our client only needs to use one hand to brush his teeth and since it is generally easier to play the drum with one hand than with two, we will focus on playing the drum with the client's dominant hand. The task analysis for the task of grasping the stick and playing the drum might be as follows:

1) Allow stick to be placed on hand;
2) Wrap fingers around stick;
3) Close fingers around stick;
4) Turn hand over so that hand is on top of (held) stick;
5) Raise hand;
6) Lower hand and stick quickly onto drum surface, without losing grip on drumstick;

7) Let drumstick come off of drum quickly or bounce off of drum, while still maintaining grasp;
8) Repeat steps 5 through 7 more than once.

It may be useful to look at some other examples of music therapy task analyses to prepare for doing your own. Hanser (1999) presents a task analysis of the steps necessary for a child to be able to perform the movements to the song "Head, Shoulders, Knees, and Toes" (pp. 173–174). Boyle and Krout (1987) present two task analyses, one for the courteous selection of partners for a movement activity and the other for playing I and V7 on the harmonica (pp. 19–25). Martin (2012) also discusses the example of supporting a client in learning how to brush their teeth, emphasizing the value of incorporating the steps into a customized song composition, allowing for practice and generalization. McLaughlin and Adler (2015) describe a case in which the music therapist completed a task analysis in collaboration with a school nurse for a child who needed frequent blood pressure readings but was fearful of the procedure. Creating a lyric substitution (also referred to as song transformation) for a familiar, favored song and then recording it facilitated not only a reduction in anxiety but also an increase in initiation and independence with the procedure.

Skill Analysis

The client must have the skills required to complete the steps in the task analysis in order for it to be appropriate. A skills analysis is done in order to identify the prerequisite skills needed to perform the tasks.

If the client does not have the skills required for the steps in the task analysis, then that particular task analysis is not useful, and it would be better to focus on a different task. In the tooth brushing example above, the client must be able to do certain things in order for the task analysis as presented to be useful. If the client is unable to coordinate grasping the toothbrush in one hand while squeezing the toothpaste onto the bristles with the other, establishing a goal for that person to brush their teeth independently would be setting him or her up for frustration and failure. It would be more appropriate to start by working on strengthening grasp and improving bilateral hand coordination. This example illustrates the value of the assessment process in developing appropriate goals and objectives and then successfully presenting tasks in therapy.

In order to be able to accomplish the steps in the task analysis for learning to brush one's teeth, it would be important to determine whether the client had adequate grasping skills, intentionality or goal-directed behavior, receptive language skills to understand instructions, fine motor coordination for moving the toothbrush in the mouth, attention skills needed to participate in instruction, and retention skills needed to remember the sequence. If these skills are not there, you need to establish the prerequisite skills before using a task approach to teaching the sequence of behaviors.

Level of Development

The third approach that is relevant to determining appropriate procedures for a music therapy session is the client's level of development. Information on developmental level is presented in Chapter 12, Further Considerations in Planning, and much of our discussion of this area will be covered when we reach that chapter. For now, though, let us say that utilizing a developmental approach in music therapy means that the therapist seeks to identify the developmental stage at which the client is functioning by comparing the client's skills to the diverse musical tasks or competencies demonstrated by normal children at each stage. For many children with delayed or atypical development, the developmental level will be uneven or will lag behind the normal skills for that chronological age. Developmental level can be applicable to clients of all ages. Developmental levels also apply to adults, both those who have delayed development and those who experience regression in old age.

Once the client's developmental level is known, two things can be done in planning. First, the next skills to be learned in normal development can be the focus of the music therapy sessions. Second, musical tasks typically done by children at that developmental level can be used with the client, since they are likely to be both engaging and useful for building the necessary skills.

The Next Step

The culmination of all of the preparation that you have been doing is the music therapy session itself. What actually occurs in the session is the focus of much of the therapist's energy. Some sessions are planned carefully in advance, and deviations from the plan occur only when necessary in order to meet client's needs. One thing to emphasize about a session that has been this carefully planned is that the planning is only for what you expect will occur. There must always be room for changes in the plan. These may occur because different clients come to the session than were expected, because they come in different moods or frames of mind than anticipated, or because something comes up in the session that calls for a change of plans. The ability to accommodate changes in the plan is essential, and the more skillful the therapist is in adapting to these changes, the more effective his or her work will be, resulting in greater success for the client(s).

The approach to some sessions is more spontaneous and can be thought of as a *structured looseness.* Although the therapist still has certain guidelines and boundaries for what is expected and acceptable and anticipated outcomes for the session are defined, the actual sequencing and structure of the session and tasks within it may be more fluid in nature. Often the clients may have goals for decision-making, choice-making, and assuming independence and responsibility. In these cases, the therapist may actually defer the planning in order to preserve these opportunities for the clients.

Music therapists working in both structured and spontaneous modes remain focused on the goals and objectives established for the clients and are aware of how the clients are doing in working toward those goals.

There is no single way to organize a music therapy session. Nonetheless, many therapists follow a basic three-part sequence: (a) some type of warm-up or introductory experience, (b) one or more experiences comprising the main part of the session, and (c) a closing or wrap-up experience. Following this structure provides a dependable framework that can be comforting to clients, can contribute to the meaning of the therapy session, and can help the therapist to achieve consistent outcomes.

The opening experience serves to bring participants (including the therapist) together by allowing them to state who they are, to share something about their mood or state of mind, and to begin to focus on the tasks and goals ahead. While music therapists sometimes call this a "hello song," this is a misnomer. The opening does not need to be a song and certainly does not need to say hello. While a song is often used as part of the opening, the opening may also include an improvisation or verbal introduction. It often includes an opportunity to find out how participants are feeling or for them to share something from their week. The opening time may provide an opportunity for the music therapist to provide an overview of the purpose of music therapy or of the session ahead, if appropriate.

The main portion of the session is where the primary work occurs. This section is composed of whatever the therapist or clients select. It is normally the longest part of the session and may include various combinations of improvising, performing or re-creating, composing, and receptive experiences. These are described in detail in Chapters 8–11.

The closing or wrap-up experience provides closure. This may be a musical closing and, as with the opening experience, may be consistent from session to session. It is often structured to provide a time for clients to share what they have gained from the session or how they are feeling at that time. It may include verbal or musical communication. The therapist should allow enough time before the scheduled end of session for all participants to express themselves so that they can move on with their day.

Setting Up the Environment

There are a number of decisions that the music therapist makes concerning the room arrangement, the equipment and instruments to be used, and materials to have on hand. Considering the consequences of these decisions ahead of time will help to ensure that the session stays focused on issues that need to be addressed and not on logistical problems.

Room Arrangement

There are several considerations regarding room arrangement. The first is the arrangement of the chairs. An arrangement in a circle or semicircle facilitates interaction, as group members will then be able to see one another. Occasionally, it works well to sit around a table. This has the advantage of allowing materials to be placed on the table, but the disadvantage is that the table becomes a barrier, physically and psychologically. In addition, tables make it more difficult for the music therapist or any assistants to move from person to person. There may be occasions in which rows work well, particularly if people need to be able to see something on the wall such as a chart or an illustration. However, sitting in rows does not promote interaction, so this arrangement should be used with caution. Regardless of the seating arrangement that you determine is most appropriate for your particular clients and purposes, be mindful that you allow adequate space for those who may be dependent on wheelchairs or other supportive mobility devices (such as walkers) to be fully included in the session.

The seating arrangement is just as important when preparing for an individual session. Consider whether the client needs special positioning in order to facilitate increased eye contact with the therapist or to allow the therapist to easily provide physical assistance to the client. Are there concerns about close physical proximity that could create anxiety for the client? If the client is dependent on a wheelchair for mobility, be sure that there is adequate space for the wheelchair to be positioned without it becoming a barrier to contact with the therapist or with instruments.

Once the decision about the room arrangement is made, it is important to be sure that the arrangement occurs. This requires that the music therapist allow time prior to the session to be sure that chairs and equipment are in place and other necessary items have been prepared. There should room for people to move around or in and out of the room, as needed. Everything should be ready when the clients begin to arrive. (There may be an occasion in which part of the therapy is for clients to assist in setting up the room. This would be a special situation and is certainly acceptable, if it serves a clinical purpose.)

After people have arrived for a group, the room arrangement may still require attention. Decide what to do with empty chairs. It is often a good idea to remove the empty chairs, since leaving them where they are contributes to a sense that the group is not complete or is not as unified as it might be. Of course, additional members may arrive later, and the music therapist needs to decide whether to add chairs when they come or leave empty chairs to be available for them. It is recommended that this decision be made consciously and with regard for its impact rather than due to convenience or lack of thought.

Equipment and Instruments

Equipment that may be needed in the music therapy session includes a piano or keyboard, other musical instruments, music stands, and a stereo/compact disc player or other equipment for accessing recorded music such as an iPod or iPad. As with the setup of the room, this needs to be planned in advance, both to ensure that they are available and so that they can be strategically placed around the room.

Music therapists also use many other instruments. There are reasons that they might choose them and considerations in using them. Some of these instruments are variations of instruments used in orchestras and bands, often simplified for music therapy as well as classroom music purposes. A good way to get an overview of the instruments that are available is to look through a catalog from a supplier that serves music therapists. You can identify these companies by accessing a conference program or searching the Web. It is also beneficial to visit the exhibit hall at a music therapy conference, where you have the opportunity to see and often play a variety of instruments as well as review printed music and other materials and resources. We will discuss instruments by category.

Pianos and keyboards. The decision about whether to use a piano or keyboard may depend on availability. But if the music therapist has the option of choosing one or the other, it is good to consider the benefits and drawbacks of each. They are not equivalent instruments. The piano has a unique sound and provides a *traditional sound for accompaniment.* It is also very substantial and may be useful when the music therapist is playing along with one or more clients. Pianos may be difficult to move and need to be kept in good condition and tuned regularly. Electronic keyboards come in various types. One advantage of a keyboard is that it is portable and can be taken to other rooms or floors; a keyboard may also be placed close to a client. Some keyboards can be programmed with various sounds, rhythms, and so forth, and some of these features may be helpful in the music therapy session. Keyboards may be programmed to provide an accompaniment, to sound like a variety of different instruments, to repeat a phrase, and for a myriad of other features. It is often a good idea to have a stand for the keyboard. Disadvantages of keyboards are that they come in a variety of sizes and types, and the music therapist needs to be familiar with the particular keyboard that is available. Some keyboards have small keys; others do not have an entire keyboard and may be missing low or high notes that the therapist needs. If batteries are used, it is important to be sure that they are fresh. It is always a good idea to have a backup set of batteries or an adapter in case the batteries lose their power. Using a cord and an adapter eliminates the need for batteries but limits the mobility of the keyboard and may be a hazard for people to trip over. The final point to keep in mind about using a keyboard is that it is *not a piano.* Use the keyboard when a keyboard is most appropriate and a piano when a piano is needed.

Accompanying and chordal instruments. This category includes pianos and keyboards, discussed above, and guitars, ukuleles, autoharps, and Qchords®. Guitars and ukuleles can be used for accompaniment and can also be taught (sometimes in simplified form) to music therapy clients. Autoharps and Qchords® are useful in that they can be placed over the laps of the therapist and client or otherwise put between them, leading to a shared experience. Autoharps must be kept in tune and time must be allotted for this. The Qchord®, a digital instrument developed by the Suzuki Company which is shaped somewhat like an autoharp, has a number of features that make it useful, including allowing for the continued playing of an accompaniment once started (when programmed to do so) and providing a satisfying musical experience with little effort.

Drums. There are many types of drums, and they have various uses. They may be played with simple or very complex rhythms. Drums make a variety of sounds, and this variety can contribute to the sound of the ensemble or composition. Some can be tuned to various pitches. Some are played with the hand, with various sounds achieved with different hand positions, while others are played with sticks or mallets. One advantage of a drum is that it can be played by almost anyone. Some drums, called hand drums or frame drums, are held in one hand, in the lap, between the legs, or under the arm. Others are placed on the floor. Some floor drums require stands; it is important that such stands be sturdy and fit the instrument properly. Since drumming can be very loud, the music therapist should be aware that people have different levels of sensitivity to sound. It is therefore a good idea to have earplugs available for clients who might like to use them and to make certain that earplugs are not shared between clients, as this could result in cross-contamination. Remo Not So Loud (NSL) drums and mallets offer another strategy for protecting the hearing of clients and therapists alike.

Sticks and mallets. Both drums and melodic percussion instruments (such as the xylophone) are played with sticks and mallets. A mallet has a covering on the end, while a stick does not. There are a number of considerations in selecting and using sticks and mallets. The head of a mallet makes a difference in the sound, so it is important to test the mallet on the selected instrument. Several mallets may be needed to produce different sounds. Most instruments are usually played with two sticks or mallets, but there are situations in which only one should be used. One of these would be when a child is just beginning to play the instrument or does not yet have the coordination necessary to use both sticks. Another would be when the player is not physically able to use both hands, perhaps due to a stroke or other injury or accident or due to a birth defect. Some instruments, such as resonator bells, are intended to be played with only one stick. Small children will require shorter sticks than larger children or adults. Finally, there will be instances in which the end of the stick that is held needs to be made larger or otherwise adapted to the needs of the person playing, and some clients can benefit from weighted mallets or mallets that are strapped to their hands or wrists.

Additional percussion instruments. There are many percussion instruments in addition to drums. Some of these are from Latin or African traditions. Some are orchestral instruments that have been adapted by music therapists. Some are simple classroom instruments. They make a variety of sounds and require varying levels of skill, although most can be played very simply.

Melodic percussion. Melodic percussion are melodic instruments that are played with a mallet or stick. Some of the finest-quality instruments have been developed for use in Orff Schulwerk and are often referred to as *Orff instruments*. They include glockenspiels (small instruments with metal bars), metallophones (with softer metal bars), and xylophones (with rosewood bars). Each of these types of instruments comes in several ranges, often soprano, alto, tenor, and bass. The bars for these Orff instruments are placed on a frame but can be taken off easily. This allows for only some of the notes to be included and is often done so that a pentatonic or other scale may be used. A bar of the same type as on the metallophone or xylophone, but in a low range, may be put on an individual frame and is called a *resonator* bar.

A pentatonic marimba is similar to the melodic instruments just described, but not part of the Orff tradition. The bars, which cannot be removed, are arranged in a pentatonic scale. This can be useful when a portable instrument is needed, for instance, when it is to be played from a hospital bed. Small xylophones that do not come from the Orff tradition are also available, but the bars will not be removable and they are generally not of the same fine quality. There may be situations, though, in which these less expensive instruments are preferred.

A xylimba is similar in that the bars cannot be removed, but it is available in a variety of pitch ranges and scales. In addition to benefits mentioned earlier regarding pitched, barred instruments which do not have removable bars (such as ease of transport), it can also be beneficial when working with clients who may intentionally or unintentionally use too much force to play instruments with removable bars. A traditional African instrument which is similar in nature is the baliphone.

Another type of melodic percussion instrument is a resonator bell or tone bar. These are individual bars that generally come in a set. One or more bars can be assigned to an individual client or to each group member. They are generally placed on a table in front of the player or may be held. Holders are available if several of these are to be used by the same person.

Several instruments have been developed that are hit with a beater built into the instrument. Handbells are the largest and most expensive of these. These are the same handbells used in churches; they have a rich, vibrant sound. They are, however, expensive and heavy and require special care; for the most part, they have been replaced in music therapy by other instruments, primarily tone chimes made by Suzuki and other companies. Both of these have good sounds and can be played by people with only one functional hand.

Wind instruments. There are a number of simple wind instruments. These include recorders, which require some skill in order to play but are within the reach of many music therapy clients. A simpler but somewhat similar instrument is a tonette.

Several instruments do not require any finger movements. These include kazoos and slide whistles. Different notes on the kazoo are made with the lips and breath. Slide whistles require modest two-hand coordination.

Single reed horns were developed largely for use with Nordoff-Robbins music. Each of these horns has a place to insert a reed that is tuned to one note, giving the therapist control over the notes that are played. Bird calls are used in some Nordoff-Robbins music, in addition to elsewhere. They are unique instruments that can be enjoyable to play.

Electronic instruments. A rapidly increasing number of electronic instruments is available. An advantage of these is that clients with a variety of physical limitations may play them or use them in other ways, such as composing. Many adaptations can be made to accommodate such limitations. For example, a switch may be devised to allow a person to select notes without having the fine motor coordination normally required to play a keyboard. Other adaptations may be similar to or modeled after those described in the next paragraph.

Adaptive instruments or materials. It is important to be aware of the physical abilities and limitations of your clients and to be prepared to provide special instruments or adapt instruments so each client can have a successful instrumental experience. A variety of adaptive instruments is described by Clark and Chadwick (1979) in *Clinically Adapted Instruments for the Multiply Handicapped*. Many adaptive instruments can be viewed and purchased through www.adaysworkmusiceducation.com. These include adaptive instrument stands, wheelchair clips for paddle drums, Velcro straps, and so on. Sometimes adapting an instrument is simply a matter of trying a variety of positioning options, but you may find that you are working with some clients who need a more individualized approach. For example, you may have a client who can produce strong tones on a reed horn but is unable to grasp it, or perhaps you are working with someone who can maintain a steady beat on a drum with his or her hand but is unable to grasp a mallet or stick. Be creative in your approach to such situations. Depending on the setting in which you are working, you may have access to occupational and physical therapists or adaptive equipment specialists who can fabricate materials for your use, or you may decide to adapt some equipment on your own. The most important thing to keep in mind is that it is your responsibility, as the therapist, to facilitate success for your clients.

Tablets, portable computers, and music players. Technology is changing rapidly, and music therapists have embraced the use of these new devices in sessions in many ways. Learning to work with digital equipment and the applications and software available is essential to music therapy treatment. Resources that enhance music-making, such as virtual sheet music and lead sheets, learning applications, and portable recording options, can supplement the use of traditional resources. A collection of electronic resources for work with children can be found in Kern (2012) while several writings outline use with adults across the life span (Knight & LaGasse, 2012; Magee et al., 2011). Useful information is also available in *Music Technology in Therapeutic and Health Settings* (Magee, 2014).

Materials

A wide variety of materials can be used in music therapy sessions. These may include song sheets, charts that are hung on the wall, and books of music.

Song sheets. A number of things need to be considered when song sheets are needed for the session. One is whether the people in the session will be able to read them. Many people, particularly older adults, cannot see without glasses and may not have glasses or cannot see well enough to read even with glasses. Many children are still in the process of learning to read or have disabilities that prevent them from being able to read song sheets. Some people for whom English is not their native language may have difficulty reading English, although they might be able to read well in their native language. In addition, it is always possible that people in the session never learned to read.

Another consideration is whether song sheets are needed for the songs being sung. If the songs are very familiar, people may not need song sheets. If that is the case, it is probably better not to use song sheets, as they will add unnecessary clutter to the session. In many cases, though, people will not be able to sing the songs from memory, so song sheets or ready-made books that include the songs should be provided. While books that include the desired songs in an acceptable format are obviously the simplest to use, there will be times when the music therapist will prefer making song sheets in order to include the necessary qualities and songs.

It is important to keep in mind that the song sheets should be helpful and not distracting. Consider having the sheets laminated and/or provided to the client with some sort of support (such as on a clipboard or specially positioned music stand) to ensure that it enhances the experience and contributes to success.

For clients who do not read music, there is no reason to have the notes included on song sheets, and song sheets that include only words are easier to type and less cumbersome to use. The words should be typed using a typeface that is large enough and dark enough for the people to read. Remember when typing that the spacing of the lines helps to guide the singer through the song; in other words, begin new lines on separate lines of the song, leave space between verses, and so forth. It is also recommended that song sheets be kept together in one book, with the pages clearly labeled.

Charts. There are a number of uses for charts in music therapy sessions. These charts may be hung on a wall or board so that clients can see them, or the information can be projected onto a screen. Sometimes words of a song will be written on a chart rather than on a song sheet. Or the chart may include an instrumental arrangement, possibly in a simplified form. We will discuss some practical aspects of making and using charts.

The main issues around chart use are similar to those with song sheets: Be sure that the people involved will be able to see and comprehend the chart and that a chart is the best way to present the material. One advantage to a chart is that it allows the therapist to direct everyone's attention to the same place, thus focusing and holding people's attention. This can be important in helping members of a group to work together. (When the same material is presented on a song sheet, the therapist has little ability to help each group member focus or keep track of where to sing or play.) However, the room or seating arrangement may not allow everyone to see the chart, and this needs to be considered beforehand. Another consideration is the amount of material to be included on the chart. Too much material may suggest that a piece of music is too complex to be contained on a single chart and is therefore too complicated for the music therapy setting.

Once the decision has been made to use a chart, the chart needs to be made so that it will be useful and visible to everyone. It must be large enough for clients to see; any lines and colors must be clear enough to be seen, and the organization must be clear.

It is a good idea to invest in some large pieces of tag board or very heavy paper. Sometimes these must then be taped together to make a large enough chart. A good way to determine the size of the tag board that is needed is to think through or write out what will be included on the chart and then buy accordingly. Writing out what will be on the chart is a good way to plan the spacing; it is certainly easier to make changes on a paper draft than on a large piece of tag board.

Evaluating Music Therapy Procedures

Following the music therapy session, the therapist will, of course, evaluate how well the client was able to perform the activities that were presented. This is accomplished using data collection/measurement systems (which may be in written, audio, or video formats) and narrative notes. More information can be found in the Documentation Strategies chapter.

It is also helpful to evaluate the effectiveness of the procedures used in the session. Just as you look at the client's success in achieving the objectives, you want to look at your success in presenting appropriate strategies for working on them. There are a number of ways to do this. All of these involve self-reflection as well as reflecting on the session and the client's response to what was presented.

It is recommended that you go through every portion of your session and evaluate both the client's response and your own reaction to what you did. In evaluating the client's response, consider how the client responded emotionally and whether it appeared that he or she enjoyed the experience, as well as how successful he or she was in accomplishing what was expected.

Assignments—Planning and Implementing Music Therapy Strategies

Consider the following to increase your understanding of session planning and implementation:

- Select a simple musical task on which you can perform a task analysis. If possible, make this something that the individual or an individual in the group with which you are working could use. Examples would be to play a drum with one stick or make a sound on a kazoo. Write a task analysis of the steps leading to being able to do this.

- Do a skills analysis of the skills needed to perform the task that you analyzed in the question above. Write out the developmental skills that you see as necessary in order for a person to do the task from your task analysis; this will have much in common with the skill analysis. How does looking at the client's skills versus developmental level inform your understanding of the client?

- Reflect on a session you recently observed or in which you participated with a music therapist. What decisions do you believe the therapist in charge of the session made regarding the room arrangement for the session? How does the arrangement vary from week to week, or how have you noticed it evolving over the time? What effects have you seen from various arrangements? Discuss these with the therapist.

- Consider the equipment and materials used in sessions at your current practicum site. How are these equipment and materials chosen? What impact might it have to introduce a different musical instrument or a different prop into the session? Were there some cases in which, upon reflection, you wish you had made different choices? If so, why? What effects have you seen from different equipment and instruments?

- Use the form "Guidelines for Activity Planning" to assist in planning for one of your sessions.

8 Improvising Experiences

This is the first of four chapters about the types of music experiences that may take place during a music therapy session. The focus of these chapters is not on specific music experiences or interventions, as these are available in other resources in the music therapy literature. The intent here is instead to present general ideas and comments on variations of music experiences.

Improvising happens when the client makes up music vocally, instrumentally, or with any body part or medium that is available, individually or with others (duet or group). The therapist helps the client to structure the experience and may improvise with the client or guide in other ways. Goal areas may include developing nonverbal means of communication and self-expression, exploring self in relation to others, stimulating the senses, and developing perceptual and cognitive skills (Bruscia, 2014b).

Variations of improvising experiences include: *instrumental nonreferential,* in which the client improvises on an instrument without reference to anything other than the music; *instrumental referential,* where the improvising is guided to represent something (such as a person, a feeling, an event, etc.); *song improvisation,* where the client spontaneously creates lyrics, melody, and/or accompaniment (this is most effective when undertaken as a solo experience); *vocal nonreferential improvisation,* in which the client improvises a vocal piece without words or images; *body improvisations,* where the client improvises with a variety of body percussion such as finger snapping, hand clapping, etc.; *mixed media improvisations,* where the client improvises using a variety of resources, including voice, body percussion, and instruments; and *conducted improvisations,* where the client creates or directs an improvisation by cuing others (Bruscia, 2014b).

Many excellent resources on improvisation and improvisation in music therapy are available. Bruscia's *Improvisational Models of Music Therapy* (1987) gives a comprehensive overview of various models of music therapy that use improvisation. Books that we recommend that can help develop skills for music therapy improvisation include some using Nordoff-Robbins resources, particularly *Creative Music Therapy* (Nordoff & Robbins, 2007) and *Healing Heritage: Paul Nordoff Exploring the Tonal Language of Music* (Robbins & Robbins, 1998). Wigram's (2004) *Improvisation: Methods and Techniques for Music Therapy Clinicians, Educators, and Students* is a very useful resource for learning to improvise. Aigen's (1998) *Paths of Development in Nordoff-Robbins Music Therapy,* which includes cases from the work of Nordoff and Robbins along with recordings of the music, provides a wealth of examples and inspiration. Gardstrom's (2007) *Music Therapy Improvisation for Groups: Essential Leadership Competencies* applies improvisation to groups, where many music therapists will use it. Another valuable resource is *Improvising in Styles: A Workbook for Music Therapists, Educators, and Musicians* (Lee & Houde, 2010), although this is quite an advanced workbook and is not recommended for your initial foray into clinical improvisation. Numerous other resources to read and learn about music therapy improvisation are available—check the websites of music therapy publishers and various music therapy journals. It is important to understand that clinical improvisation doesn't just happen. It is a skill that must be practiced and honed, just like other clinical skills and techniques.

Children with Special Needs

Using improvising experiences with children with special needs can be especially valuable in helping the therapist discover what types of music and instruments are motivating and stimulating for the children. This makes improvisation particularly useful for assessment. Due to the developmental level of most children with special needs, these experiences will most often be nonreferential. An example of instrumental nonreferential improvisation would be to present a child with a standing drum and a pair of mallets and allow him or her to initiate playing the music without providing modeling or instructions. This can uncover information about sensorimotor skills (grasp, bilateral coordination), cognitive concepts (imitation or repetition of patterns), communication skills (turn-taking or continuous beating), affective/emotional development and self-regulation (playing musically or using the drum to make noise), and much more. Engaging in improvisation can help a child with autism, who may have difficulty with transitions or changes. The therapist may initially follow the child's improvising and gradually try to introduce changes to help the child better organize his or her responses. Similar strategies and outcomes can be achieved with vocal nonreferential improvisations as well. Body improvisations can also provide a stimulating experience for a child. Improvisation in therapy can also be an invaluable tool for evaluation through providing a way to measure various musical responses and their development over time.

Adolescents and Adults with Intellectual and Developmental Disabilities

Improvising experiences in therapy with adolescents and adults with developmental disabilities facilitates the development of nonverbal communication and expression of emotion. Even for clients who have verbal skills, the opportunity to express themselves through improvisation may be less threatening than talking. Improvisation provides an expanded range of expression, while using words often limits communication. In a group setting, improvisational experiences can enhance the opportunities for developing relationships with other group members as a result of the musical development over time. Group improvisation heightens feelings of belonging and productivity through contributing to a group undertaking. It also provides natural opportunities for group members to experiment with leadership roles as well as to practice turn-taking, sharing, and following, such as through conducted improvisations.

Adults with Psychiatric Disorders

Improvising experiences for adults with psychiatric disorders serve many purposes. These experiences may be used to help a client who is experiencing a psychotic episode focus on the external here-and-now reality or to assist a person in crisis in expressing the emotional trauma nonverbally. Improvisation experiences ranging from structured to free and from referential to nonreferential have been used with this population.

A simple improvising experience for a group involves presenting a variety of instruments and asking each participant to choose one. Group members are first instructed to listen to a free improvisation begun by a volunteer or the group member with the instrument the therapist has identified as the lead instrument (e.g., the alto xylophone). Group members are then invited to join the improvisation by adding a sound when they feel ready. As the music unfolds, the therapist's role can be small or large. This is a time when the therapist's sensitivity to the clients' music is very important, as group members are given the freedom to create but offered enough musical support from the therapist to work together. Should the group be unable to work together with or without the therapist's guidance, this can be discussed after the experience. Group members may be asked to reflect on how they listen, how they work with others, how they respond to the unexpected, and how they interact in uncomfortable situations, as well as consider other relationship issues arising from this experience. A simple improvisation may become the focus of an entire session as group members explore verbally, and then improvisationally, how they relate to one another through the music.

More complex improvisational experiences can be created through the use of ensemble. Members are assigned specific parts to play for a portion of the improvisation, while a solo or duet is created improvisationally, either over the group ensemble or in designated places within the structure of the music. This form of improvisation can be referential, although it is most often nonreferential. This style of improvisation requires the therapist to assume more responsibility for structuring the musical experience. While group members need not provide as much organization for the music, the improvisers are provided with a smaller and tighter structure within which to work. The therapist may find this type of improvisation useful for clients who need more help in organizing their external world.

Older Adults with Age-Related Needs

To create a referential instrumental improvisation for a group of older adults, the therapist might ask members to select simple percussive and melodic instruments and then work with the group to establish a theme (perhaps related to an upcoming holiday or season or an emotion) and perform a referential improvisation based on that theme. This could be followed by a discussion of the feelings elicited by the improvisation, including associations and memories related to the theme. A theme of *springtime,* for instance, is likely to elicit memories and feelings of spring. Substituting the use of voices for the instruments could create a vocal improvisation. Similarly, the use of various body parts could create a body improvisation, and combining more than one medium in the improvisation could lead to a mixed media improvisation. The music therapist's role would be to facilitate the improvisation and might include playing with the clients.

A nonreferential instrumental improvisation would follow a similar format but without specifying a theme. The improvisation in this case would be music for its own sake without reference to anything outside of the music. The discussion that follows could focus on feelings about the music and the experience. As with the referential improvisation, nonreferential improvisation can be adapted for use with vocals, body parts, or mixed media. In structuring a nonreferential improvisation, the therapist may offer anything from very little to quite a lot of direction, depending upon the abilities of the group members.

Improvisation may also be used with individuals. The therapist may invite the client to use either the referential or nonreferential format to meet a wide range of goals. For example, the therapist may ask the client to improvise the sound of a specific emotion (referential) or may ask the client to play whatever he or she would like (nonreferential). The therapist may then intensify the experience by entering into the improvisation musically with the client or may engage the client in a discussion of the process.

People in Medical Settings

Most acutely ill medical patients are seen individually, often in a hospital room. This creates some logistical issues, as there may be a roommate or a person in the room next door who may also be affected by the music experience. Special attention should be given to the needs of those in close proximity to the patient when planning for music therapy interventions. This may mean including the roommate in the session, modifying the session so as not to disturb the other person, moving to an alternate space for the session (with physician approval), or even not having the session if there is no way to avoid disturbing the other person in the room.

Medical patients often experience a wide range of emotions and physical symptoms. Offering an experience in which the patient is able to give musical sound to the pain, anxiety, or sadness associated with illness and hospitalization can be very effective. Keeping in mind that improvisation may be unfamiliar to the patient, the therapist might offer a few selected musical instruments with which to work—perhaps an ocean drum, glockenspiel, pentatonic marimba, autoharp, or Qchord®. All of these instruments can be used with minimal instruction, and each offers a different type of musical experience. The improvisation may be referential ("play the pain"), or it may be more open ("play whatever you need to express or say in the music"). Following the music, the therapist may wish to process the experience verbally or may use more music or a related art experience such as drawing to assist the patient in working with the material expressed in the music.

Note that the improvisation experiences suggested for older adults and people in medical settings have some similarities; these suggestions may also be similar to those for the other client groups that have been described. This is because all people share the basic need to express emotions. Improvisations may also be fruitfully used to meet unique needs of these populations.

Uses in the Music Therapy Literature
Children with Special Needs

The pioneering work of Nordoff and Robbins (1971, 2007), based on clinical improvisation, led the way in the use of improvisation with children who have special needs. Many therapists have used and evolved the Nordoff-Robbins approach. One example is Robarts's (Trevarthen, Aitken, Papoudi, & Robarts, 1998) work with children with autism, which includes a case study using improvisation in the successful treatment of a child with autism. This boy was 3½ when he began music therapy. Robarts describes her work and includes the issues that were important during each stage of work, as well as her interpretation of the child's responses. This case is valuable because of the detail that it provides in using improvisation.

Paraverbal therapy, developed by Heimlich and closely related to music therapy, uses improvisation in a number of ways. Bruscia (1987) includes play improvisations, musical story improvisations, and song improvisations as employed by Heimlich (1965, 1972) and other paraverbal therapists (McDonnell, 1983; Wheeler, 1987).

Rogers (2003) described the use of improvisation in working with an 11-year-old girl who was in the foster care system. She says, "Music therapy is a particularly useful therapeutic modality for work with abused clients as it specifically offers the opportunity to explore and express feelings that the child may find difficult or may be unable to verbalize" (p. 128). During a 55-session therapy sequence, the girl moved from being anxious about her playing and restricted in her improvisations to being able to "express a wide range of emotions ... ranging from sadness to joy, from despair to delight ... [and] developed more individuated self-expression, developing a new sense of self, creativity, and autonomy" (p. 134).

Improvisation can be used with groups of children as well as individuals. Carter and

Oldfield (2002) describe their use of a structured improvisation in which children are encouraged to "play freely" while the piano plays, then stop when the piano stops. Oldfield (Oldfield & Bunce, 2001) also used improvisation with a group of mothers and young children. Many more excellent accounts of work with children with special needs can be found in *Case Examples of Improvisational Music Therapy,* edited by Bruscia (2014a).

Adolescents and Adults with Intellectual and Developmental Disabilities

Watson (2002) describes an improvisational approach with a woman with severe developmental disabilities. The goal of the sessions was to "experience affective musical contact with the therapist" (p. 105). To accomplish this, the music therapist used her voice and a metallophone to contact the client. Watson does not include an entire case study but rather small segments from the work with detailed analyses of what occurred in the sessions. Because of these detailed analyses, this case can provide a rich understanding of what can occur in an improvisational session with a person with severe disabilities.

Boxill (1985) describes the use of "Our Contact Song," which she describes as "a composed or improvised song that lends itself to improvisational changes and adaptations. It becomes a fountainhead for a myriad of activities and experiences, always changing and being transformed in the service of therapeutic goals" (p. 81). This song, which is often improvised, is a cornerstone of Boxill's approach. She says, "Our Contact Song is the first reciprocal musical expression, the first two-way musical communication, the first overt musical indication *initiated by the client* of an awareness of the existence of another" (p. 80).

Aigen (2002) illustrates the use of popular musical styles in Nordoff-Robbins clinical improvisation with a nonverbal man with a developmental delay when beginning the music therapy process at 27 years of age. Aigen describes the course of this man's therapy over a number of years, using popular musical idioms for the improvisational music therapy process. Aigen connects what is happening musically with the goals that are being met through the music. This example is published with an accompanying CD featuring the musical examples described in the book.

Also using the Nordoff-Robbins approach, Turry and Marcus (2003) worked with a group of four adult clients with diagnoses on the autism spectrum. They describe two methods used: realization (the use of precomposed pieces) and improvisation. Their description of the work of this group is very informative, as they show its progress through different stages of development and also include significant moments for the members, in each case including both musical and interpersonal information that makes the session come alive to the reader.

Similarly, Aigen (1997) describes the work of four adolescents with various developmental disabilities over the course of a year in a creative music therapy group, with an emphasis on the development of songs and thematic material that evolved out of spontaneous improvisations. Detailed descriptions of conversation and interaction amongst the clients and therapists are interwoven with musical notation of emerging song structures. A companion video that allows the reader to view session excerpts is also available.

Adults with Psychiatric Disorders

Many examples of using improvisation with adults with psychiatric disorders are available. A book by Borczon (1997) contains several examples of the use of improvisation with adults in treatment for chemical dependency and/or psychiatric difficulties. One example (Chapter 6), concerning a group of adults in treatment for chemical dependency, is a session in which he told a story while having the group members participate in the story musically by improvising. He then helped the group members to relate to themes that grew from the story. Many of their responses allowed them to go deeply into feelings that they needed to work with and express.

Adults in acute psychiatric treatment in a short-term hospital unit used improvisation to express unnamed emotions and bring them to consciousness (Shultis, 1999). Group members were also asked to play an instrument to reflect their current emotional state; other group members offered feedback describing the music or the emotional quality of the sound. The improviser could gain insight into the expressed emotions when hearing it described by others or might find words to more accurately describe the emotion that was previously felt but not consciously owned.

Sadovnik (2014) used rap and hip-hop to address the needs of patients in an adult inpatient psychiatric unit. He discusses the development of a program that included a recording studio. He describes work with a 28-year-old patient with schizophrenia who had trouble liking or accepting his improvisations. The client was able to work with a song that included the phrases "I can't" and "I'm designed to win, not to lose" and, after considerable work, made it into a song that he felt good about and that expressed his feelings. He was given a CD of the song and was encouraged to listen to it nonjudgmentally, as he had composed it.

Another example of the use of improvisation with adults is in Analytical Music Therapy, developed by Mary Priestley. While Analytical Music Therapy requires special training beyond the basic music therapy training, music therapy students should be familiar with this approach (Eschen, 2002; Priestley, 1994; Scheiby, 2015). Another of the many available examples is the work of Austin (2008), who uses vocal improvisation in working with adults with emotional difficulties.

Older Adults with Age-Related Needs

Reuer, Crowe, and Bernstein (1999) developed a variety of group percussion strategies that can be used with older adults, with a focus on promoting wellness. They describe a number of techniques utilizing egg shakers, paddle drums, and other percussion techniques, including a number of ways to use improvisation.

Scheiby (1999) describes an adaptation of Analytical Music Therapy in a "supportive music psychotherapeutic approach" (p. 270) with a group of older adults who had mild to severe dementia and depression along with a variety of neurological problems, including strokes. The case study includes the use of improvisation to support a person feeling lonely and sad and to help other group members get in touch with their feelings.

D. Aldridge (1996) describes the use of Nordoff-Robbins–based improvisation with a woman in the early stages of Alzheimer's disease. Connections were made between the woman's playing and the characteristics of Alzheimer's, thus providing insight into the appearance and progression of the disease (pp. 197–203).

Darnley-Smith and Patey (2003) used improvisation with an older woman who had Alzheimer's disease. The woman followed the therapist closely and, if the therapist paused in the music, the client also paused, looking anxiously at the therapist. They say, "It seemed that she needed to be accompanied all the time to feel confident enough to play. After some experimenting, [the therapist] began to play a continuous, slow, walking rhythm ... in the tempo of Sheila's playing" (p. 76). They felt that the repetition of the rhythmic structure allowed the woman to continue playing and to gradually experiment with different sounds.

People in Medical Settings

Ann Turry (1997) describes the use of clinical improvisation to alleviate distress during medical procedures in young children who are hospitalized. She suggests uses of music therapy and improvisation before, during, and after medical procedures and describes considerations in using music therapy in this setting.

In an example of the use of improvisation with adults with medical problems, G. Aldridge (1996) describes the use of melodic improvisation with women with breast cancer. In addition to giving an overview of what she discovered in researching this area, she provides a case study of melodic improvisation with a woman in the week following surgery for breast cancer. Also working with adults, Gustorff (2001) describes music therapy with people who are in comas in intensive care. She generally begins by breathing in rhythm with them and then lets an improvisation flow from this rhythm. She says, "I take up the breathing rhythm, breathe with the patient, and finally sing following his rhythm (without text, vocalizing). I go to meet him musically at his current position and share with him one of his more intimate, life-giving rhythms. The singing improvisation, which develops jointly with the patient, is geared exclusively to his powers" (p. 67).

Pothoulaki, MacDonald, and Flowers (2012) studied the impact of group improvisational music therapy, based on the Nordoff-Robbins approach, with cancer patients in a day program hospice setting. The groups met twice a week for an hour over the course of six weeks. Session content included free improvisation (nonreferential), as well as more structured improvisation (referential or guided). Pitched and unpitched percussion instruments were available for the patients to access, as well as a couple of wind instruments (i.e., pan pipe and whistle). A number of recurring themes emerged over the course of therapy, with a concentration on illness, relaxation, and self-confidence. Group members experienced benefits from the opportunity to communicate nonverbally and to develop a sense of belonging by connecting with others who were experiencing similar challenges.

Considerations

As the summaries above demonstrate, there are many ways to use improvising experiences. Some people assume that improvisational experiences use only piano, always include the therapist along with the client, or follow only a particular musical style such as jazz. In actuality, many improvisations use only simple rhythm instruments, are done by a client alone or by an entire group, and utilize a variety of styles and modalities, including atonality.

Another point that may not be appreciated by the novice improviser is that most improvisation, while it may appear unstructured, does in fact depend on an underlying structure. Many a new therapist is surprised to give instruments to a group of children, for example, and ask one to play a drum, assuming that this child will keep a beat and thus provide grounding for the group—only to discover that the child has no sense of a steady beat and to watch the improvisation fall apart. Part of learning to use improvisation effectively is understanding the amount of structure that is helpful but not too controlling.

Improvisational experiences will often be combined with other music therapy experiences to form an entire session. Indeed, there may be times when a planned strategy turns into an improvisational one, to the benefit of all. In contrast, there can be instances during an improvisation when a thematic structure may emerge that, when extended and reintroduced, may develop into a song and ultimately move from being part of an improvisation to being part of a composition experience—and perhaps eventually even to being used for a re-creative experience. For example, many of the Nordoff-Robbins compositions began as in-the-moment improvisations. These compositions include simple songs, musical dramas, and ensemble music-making pieces.

Improvisational experiences are not appropriate for all clients. Deciding on the level of structure in the improvisation, or when not to use improvisation, is based on the unique needs of the client. The main considerations have to do with the abilities of the clients and what you hope to accomplish through the improvisation.

While novice therapists or improvisers can conduct improvisational music therapy sessions, improvisations can become more sophisticated and the therapist's role more important as his or her skills in improvisation and therapy increase. Facilitating a sophisticated improvisational session requires a high level of skill, particularly with some populations and in certain settings.

Materials

The most obvious materials necessary for facilitating improvising experiences are a wide variety of instruments for client use, including pitched instruments (barred instruments, tunable drums, etc.) and unpitched percussion (shakers, etc.), wind instruments (reed horns, whistles, etc.), string instruments (guitar, autoharp, etc.), and piano. Body percussion and vocal improvisation are also important experiences within improvisations. Other items can also be used—be creative! Think of the exciting music produced through the use of paper and plastic bags, brooms, trash can lids, and small cardboard gift boxes by the creators and performers of the very popular show *Stomp,* the creative use of PVC piping and other everyday items by *Blue Man Group,* and similar approaches by other performance artists. In addition, don't overlook the improvising opportunities provided by electronic instruments and computers.

People often improvise with a collection of simple rhythm and melodic instruments. In this case, it is best to select instruments with varying pitches, ranges, and timbres. However, it is important that melodic instruments be able to play in the same key. If you are using Orff xylophones or other instruments with removable bars or other pitched instruments such as reed horns, tone chimes, and so on, be sure that you prepare the instruments in the same key as the other instruments that will be used in the improvisation.

Tips for Using

There are many ways to learn to improvise. You may learn the process by experimenting with your own musical skills, by engaging in workshop and classroom sessions that teach about structuring improvisation (such as Orff training), or by improvising with clients and letting them teach you what they need from you. Wigram (2004) provides many suggestions for learning to improvise in *Improvisation: Methods and Techniques for Music Therapy Clinicians, Educators, and Students,* intended to function as a method book—a tutor, a "practice" book that gives concrete, practical examples in the text "of how to explore the potential and freedom of musical improvisation, and how to use that freedom in developing improvisational skills and then applying those skills in therapeutic interventions" (p. 23).

Basics of improvisation on the piano can be found in Humphries' (2010) *Piano Improvisation Handbook*, a volume filled with foundational exercises and a wealth of suggestions for using various harmonic progressions.

The key is to be clear about your intent and to bravely begin. It is sometimes helpful to begin with more planned procedures and introduce improvisation as a segment of a musical experience. For example, you might have a group keep a steady beat or play a simple rhythmic ostinato pattern while one player improvises over the sound. Initially, the therapist may play this improvisation as an example for the clients, or a client who is ready for this challenge may play it. You can gradually allow the ostinato players to move away from the prescribed rhythm and begin to add a sound that fits with what the improviser is playing. This will allow a group to gradually move into the improvisational experience while keeping it structured for the sake of inexperienced improvisers, therapist or clients.

Some students are intimidated by improvisation. Often, this is because they have the idea that there are rights and wrongs when improvising. While it is a good idea to practice improvising when you are away from your therapy session, it is also important to *just do it* in the session. If you just move ahead with an improvisation, with you on one instrument and your client on one or more other instruments, you will probably discover that you *can* improvise. Once you are more comfortable improvising, you can work to refine your improvisational and clinical skills.

Another misconception is that improvisations have to be complicated. They do not! You may want to begin with an improvisation in which you play a steady beat on a drum and your client plays another instrument. Many therapeutic goals can be accomplished with this kind of simple improvisation. In fact, it is not uncommon for someone just beginning to use improvisation to play too many notes in too sophisticated a manner, leaving the client to struggle to find an opportunity to join or feeling intimidated that their contributions might not be valued.

Similarly, improvisations do not have to be tonal or use a traditional Western scale. Many clinical improvisations are intentionally *not* tonal. Once again, as you progress, you will be able to build your skill in utilizing the improvisation to help your clients reach their clinical goals.

Do not assume that each client will be able to play in rhythm or that clients will necessarily play together or listen to each other as they play. These skills require a higher level of musical and interpersonal sensitivity than some clients possess. These may be part of their clinical goals, but do not be surprised if they do not occur automatically.

Finally, keep in mind that your role as a music therapist is to facilitate the improvisation. This may mean playing a basic beat or maintaining a grounding for the improvisation. It means that throughout the improvisation, you should remain aware of what is occurring with the clients, both musically and personally. When we can balance and facilitate these aspects and use improvisation to help our clients grow, improvising experiences can be very rewarding!

Assignments—Improvising Experiences

Use these assignments to deepen your understanding of how you might use improvising experiences in your music therapy work:

- Describe a time when you observed a therapist using an improvising experience (a videotape or demonstration is okay). Based on the improvising experiences suggested by Bruscia (2014b) and described in the second and third paragraphs of this chapter, are you able to identify the specific type of improvising experience that was implemented? What did you observe in the responses of the client(s) that could help the therapist determine if the experience was beneficial?
- Think about incorporating the use of an improvising experience in one of your

sessions. Would such an intervention be appropriate? What did you read that can help you to determine when it is appropriate to use improvising experiences? If you cannot answer this question, seek guidance from your instructor or site supervisor.

- Considering the goals and objectives you already have identified for your client(s), how could you structure the intervention to include an improvising experience? Which type or types of improvising experiences might be beneficial for your client(s)? How will you determine which type or types of improvising experiences to include, based on the anticipated benefits? How can you best prepare yourself to organize, present, develop, and process the experience?

- Find two examples of the use of improvising experiences with your current population in the literature; try to locate one example of use in individual therapy and another example of group work. Describe them and provide the sources.

- For the current client(s) you are observing and/or with whom you are working, ask your clinical supervisor to describe some possible applications of improvising experiences that have been or could be implemented. If improvising experiences have been used in previous sessions, how have the client(s) responded? If improvising experiences have not been used, is there a reason that they are counterindicated? Or, does your supervisor think that there could be benefits in providing such an experience? If so, are you able to participate in the development and/or presentation of an improvising experience?

9 Re-creative Experiences

In re-creative experiences, the client learns or performs precomposed music or reproduces any type of musical form presented as a model. These also include structured music experiences in which the client performs predefined roles or behaviors. In instances in which these experiences occur before an audience, the term "performing" is used, but "re-creative" is a more accurate term for clinical use. Goals may include skill development in areas such as sensorimotor, memory and recall, and time-ordered behavior; self-awareness and awareness of others; and interpersonal interaction and a sense of community (Bruscia, 2014b).

Variations of re-creating experiences include: *instrumental re-creation* (playing an instrument) or *vocal re-creation* (singing a song), in which the client plays or sings in a prescribed or written manner, thus reproducing structured or precomposed musical materials or songs; *performance,* where a client plays or sings before an audience; *musical productions,* in which the client participates in the planning and provision of a performance event; *musical games and activities,* where the client is involved in games or activities that are structured by music; and *conducting,* where the client directs the live performance of others (Bruscia, 2014b).

Children with Special Needs

Re-creative experiences can provide children with special needs with a unique opportunity to combine the development of functional skills (such as attending, memory, and sequencing skills) and academic achievement with broad enhancements in self-esteem and the development of peer relationships. For example, the client may be engaged in learning basic or adapted music notation in order to play a simple piece on resonator bells, which can simultaneously address skills in reading, math, or color identification. The client may then perform the same piece as part of a small recital experience for classmates, which also serves to enhance the child's self-image and expand how peers and teachers view him or her. The client may next transfer this skill to playing a small but pivotal percussion line in the school band concert, where he or she can interact with a much wider social circle than ever before.

Hintz (2013a), presenting information on music therapy with autistic spectrum disorder, says that singing songs "can serve a number of clinical needs, including providing opportunities for learning new information ..., practicing fundamental communication skills ..., challenging and practicing shifting attention, increasing motivation for engagement with others, and expanding repertoires of responding" (p. 70). She says, though, that "the child's need for increasing social motivation, engagement, and reciprocity" (p. 70) underlies all other intents for singing songs.

Adolescents and Adults with Intellectual and Developmental Disabilities

Re-creative experiences can produce similarly broad results with adults with intellectual and developmental disabilities. Additionally, these types of music experiences provide numerous opportunities for helping clients practice social situations and expectations within the structure of the music therapy environment and then transfer these skills to actual social settings. Examples of this include learning precomposed therapy songs that deal with personal care, social situations, or managing difficult emotions. When clients learn and internalize the song structure (melody, harmony, rhythm), they develop a tangible tool that they can access when needed. Singing preferred songs or playing musical games in a group can enhance the clients' connection to one another and build social relationships and a sense of community.

Adults with Psychiatric Disorders

Adults with psychiatric disorders may frequently be involved in creating and performing music together. This may include group singing, ensemble music-making, dancing, and solo performance. Such experiences present opportunities for clients to be themselves in a musical environment, to receive feedback from others about their performance, and to deepen their sense of competence and self-worth.

Group singing may be used as a recreational program or may be a part of a group therapy experience. Choosing songs that have meaning to the client, sharing their personal significance, and singing them with a group can all lead to a deeper sense of being understood or *heard* by others and can deepen the bonds among group members.

Rewarding music ensemble experiences may be accomplished using instruments that require little or no previous musical training. Such simple musical works such as *Fun for Four Drums* (Nordoff & Robbins, 1968a) and *A Garden of Bell Flowers* (Levin & Levin, 1977) can be performed with simple instructions from the therapist. The therapist carries the bulk of the responsibility for creating the musical portrait in sound, while the clients are responsible for contributing their musical motifs at the appropriate time. This may also help to develop reality-based *here-and-now* responses for those experiencing psychosis.

Dancing is a popular activity with adults with these difficulties, as this common social experience is not so common in the lives of many such clients. The existence of the safe environment and clear boundaries, together with the rhythm of the music, allows for an appropriate and enjoyable physical closeness that can be a powerful motivator for some clients. For clients with psychoses, dancing can work well as a reward after a more task-oriented session.

A solo performance within a group setting or as a part of a talent show is also a common use of music with this population. The music therapist often takes on the role of teacher and coach, preparing and supporting the client before, during, and after the performance. Clients reap many benefits from these experiences, including increased self-confidence, appropriate attention, and a sense of belonging to the treatment community.

Older Adults with Age-Related Needs

Sing-alongs are frequently included in music therapy with older adults and typically involve singing familiar songs. Since singing is a social activity in most cultures, it is a logical way to involve people. In addition, singing is fun! Memories or feelings elicited by the music may be processed verbally, extending the sing-along to include reminiscence and other forms of engagement.

Re-creating experiences also include songs or other compositions in which participants perform a composed part. A popular song that may be used at many ages, "The Hokey Pokey," is a good example. Re-creating experiences also include instrumental performance experiences where clients use tone chimes or percussion instruments, for example, to play specific parts of a song. Many simple songs designed for use in Orff music education can be adapted for use with older adults, as can music used in music therapy with other populations.

Older adults may also enjoy and benefit from performing music that they have known earlier in their lives. While some may not feel that they are still able to perform, they can still get great fulfillment from participating. Often, people who did not perform when they were younger may find that they enjoy it when they are older. The use of a choir format to engage clients in performance is common in long-term care facilities and offers opportunities for singing and playing instruments as well as perhaps dancing and movement to music. These performances frequently draw an audience of peers, staff, and family members and afford the older adults a boost in self-confidence and a greater sense of community within the performing group and the facility. Some music stores have promoted the opportunity for healthy older adults to learn to play instruments. Music therapists are often sought to assist with these programs because of their skill in adapting musical learning to people's individual needs.

People in Medical Settings

Medical patients are often involved in re-creative music therapy experiences through singing. Songs may be chosen as a means of self-expression, as a connection to the patient's outside world, because of their value and meaning to the patient, or because they introduce a topic or theme to be explored in the session. Singing also provides physical benefits, particularly for those with respiratory ailments, as the deep breathing required for singing can facilitate a productive cough in patients with pneumonia and chronic lung disease. Singing and deep breathing can also lead to physiological relaxation.

Simple instruments may also be used in re-creating experiences with patients in medical settings. Resonator bells or tone chimes can be used to play simple melodies. Often, each patient will be given one or two notes to play. Music can be performed by ear or by using a simple chart, or the music therapist can indicate when the patient is to play. Rhythm instruments and a Qchord® may also be useful. Not only can these experiences be musically satisfying, but also they help patients to rebuild strength they may have lost through being bedridden.

Uses in the Music Therapy Literature
Children with Special Needs

Nordoff and Robbins (1983) outline a number of uses of precomposed music for children with special needs, and Robbins and Robbins (1980) do this for children who are deaf and hard-of-hearing as well as other children. They and their colleagues have composed and published a variety of songs for work with children, including books of songs (Levin & Levin, 1997; Nordoff & Robbins, 1962, 1968b, 1980a, 1980b, 1980c, 1995), musical plays (Nordoff & Robbins, 1966, 1969), and songs with instrumental accompaniments (Levin & Levin, 1977, 1998, 2004; Nordoff & Robbins, 1968a, 1972, 1979). Additional contributions of songs and music with instrumental accompaniments to this genre of music therapy literature include *Themes for Therapy* (Ritholz & Robbins, 1999) and *More Themes for Therapy* (Ritholz & Robbins, 2002). These resources are highly recommended for people working with children, regardless of whether they use the Nordoff-Robbins approach.

Hibben (1991), working with a group of children with attention-deficit hyperactivity disorder, used the precomposed song "Frog Went A-Courtin'" in her sessions. She speaks first of how the children's reaction—teasing her for the way she said "ahummm, ahummm" at the end of each verse—indicated increasing trust of her and that she would not leave or rebuke them for this. Later, the children used this song as the basis for a musical drama. This involved dancing and later finding hiding places as part of the song. This drama required negotiation and new roles, all allowing for and indicating growth in the children.

Adolescents and Adults with Intellectual and Developmental Disabilities

Boxill (1985) describes singing an opening song in which members are acknowledged by name and involved in various ways, including playing rhythm instruments (pp. 145–150), illustrating the use of re-creative strategies using both vocal and instrumental music. She also describes the use of re-creating techniques with a 29-year-old man with moderate developmental disability who had hemiplegia and was dependent on a wheelchair for mobility (pp. 131–133). This man enjoyed the song "Guantanamera," and Boxill used it in its original form and then matched and reflected the man's drum beating. She reported that the trust and pleasure generated allowed him to begin to beat the drum in a more coordinated manner. They also used another song, "Kum ba Yah," to work on articulation.

Music Is for Everyone (Farnan & Johnson, 1988b) contains music composed especially for people with severe developmental disabilities. While the authors do not give clinical examples, the songs they provide are appropriate for both children and adults with developmental disabilities. Titles include "Pick Your Head Up," "Pick a Bell or Pick a Maraca," and "Touch the Tambourine." A second book by the same authors, *Everyone Can Move* (1988a), also contains songs composed for this population.

Some songs created for children with special needs may be easily adapted to use with adults with developmental disabilities. Much of the Nordoff and Robbins music and the instrumental and vocal pieces by Levin and Levin are ageless in their lyrical content and musical structure.

Adults with Psychiatric Disorders

Engaging people who experience psychosis in the rhythmic playing of pre-established patterns can be useful in helping to organize their thinking processes. Shultis (1999) used rhythmic drumming to focus clients' attention and found that they were often more verbally organized after playing.

Reed (2002) describes the use of a gospel choir with adults classified as mentally disordered offenders in a state hospital setting. Employing a structure that generally begins with a call-and-response warm-up song, the group then learns new material using lyric sheets, and songs are eventually memorized. Techniques are adapted to the learning level of each member. Sessions always end with the repetition of songs learned earlier in the session and a closing prayer. Reed suggests the following goals among those that may be accomplished through the gospel choir: provide an outlet for emotional expression; serve as a bridge to social participation; demonstrate an acceptance of guidance, leadership, and social feedback; attend the group on time and without prompting; and gain a new leisure skill.

Eyre (2011b) reported on a study in which adults diagnosed with major mental illness participated in a bilingual choir as part of an outpatient treatment department. Self-reports by participants indicated that they felt that self-esteem, emotional expression and mood, ability to cope with stress, comfort level within the group, and establishment of a dependable routine were the aspects of their lives that were most positively impacted by their involvement in the therapeutic choir. Clearly, universal elements of choirs—such as regular times for rehearsals, working together toward common outcomes, shared learning of various genres and elements of music, and presentation of final products—which are all integral to re-creative experiences in music therapy, hold natural, positive opportunities for those working to improve their quality of life.

Murphy (2015), discussing music therapy with people with substance abuse disorders, suggests that therapeutic sing-alongs (those that were goal-directed or focused on a theme related to recovery) could be useful in early recovery to develop group cohesion or tolerance of others. Later in treatment, she suggests that they can be used to identify and communicate feelings.

Older Adults with Age-Related Needs

Many music therapists incorporate sing-alongs into programs with older adults. Chavin (1991) finds sing-alongs helpful for people with dementia and suggests some modifications in order to meet their needs. She also offers several ideas for making sing-alongs as effective as possible. Shaw (1993) provides month-by-month examples of sing-along ideas and other experiences appropriate for holidays and seasons. Clair (1996) gives suggestions for using singing with people even into later stages of dementia but acknowledges that with the progression of dementia, clients will not be able to remember the words to many songs. She points out, though, that songs learned early in life will be retained longer than those learned later.

Clair (1996) also finds that people with dementia can do ballroom dancing quite far into their illness, especially with their spouses as partners. Others (Chavin, 1991; Gfeller & Hanson, 1995) also use dancing and other movement techniques in music therapy sessions with older people.

Dassa and Amir (2014) studied the role of singing familiar songs and its impact on encouraging conversation in people with middle- to late-stage Alzheimer's disease. Although the study was brief (six participants in a music therapy group that met eight times over the course of one month), an analysis of verbal and sung content revealed that songs from the participants' past elicited memories. Conversation related to the singing of these familiar songs was notably increased, and the experience of group singing also resulted in more spontaneous verbalization. Further, group members voiced positive feelings and showed increases in sense of accomplishment and belonging after singing.

The use of performing experiences with instruments is described frequently, often as part of a rhythm band. The use of rhythm instruments should be structured in some way. Although untrained people frequently hand clients rhythm instruments and have them play with no particular structure or goal in mind, this is not recommended. Chavin (1991) uses rhythm instruments with people who need to walk (or pace), accompanying a song that the client and therapist sing together. Gfeller and Hanson (1995) provide a number of useful ideas for structuring performing experiences by utilizing rhythm instruments. Instruments may also be used in other ways. Shaw (1993) describes the use of a bell band, in which each participant has a resonator bell and beater and plays a familiar tune when pointed to by the leader.

Clair and Memmott (2008) describe the important role that music can play in helping healthy older adults remain healthy. She points out that many older people who are healthy have the time and energy to develop or relearn musical skills. They describe a number of instances in which older adults learned or relearned musical instruments and the positive effects on self-esteem and social interaction that grew from these experiences.

Reuer, Crowe, and Bernstein (1999) describe a number of percussion-based strategies for working with older adults with a focus on promoting and maintaining wellness. Glassman (1983) organized a talent show to meet the needs of healthy older people attending a senior center. She describes the entire process from the auditions through set design and staging, culminating in the performances and the reactions of participants.

People in Medical Settings

Marley (1996) uses precomposed songs and simple musical instruments with hospitalized infants and toddlers in a child life program. She describes several techniques using precomposed songs. These songs, sung a number of times while the music therapist sways with the child, are intended to encourage a comfortable rapport between the adult and child. She also describes a rhythm band in which the child plays an instrument to the accompaniment of recorded music.

Cevasco (2014) recorded mothers singing songs that they thought the infants would hear when they came home. She reported a situation in which she recorded the mother of an infant in the neonatal intensive care unit (NICU) singing songs that she had determined she should include by asking grandparents and other family members what songs they thought they would sing to the baby. Reflecting on the mothers who had made these recordings, Cevasco says, "Mothers were often empowered at times when they felt helpless and hopeless by recording their singing to be played for their infants when they could not be visiting in the NICU. Giving parents a CD to take home provided an opportunity for parents to continue using music in the home environment" (p. 124).

Shultis and Gallagher (2015) describe a number of advantages of singing with patients who are hospitalized. An example illustrates some of the benefits:

> A family with whom the music therapist had been working for several weeks was experiencing anticipatory grief as the husband neared death. The wife, who had previously chosen to leave the room during her husband's music therapy sessions, appeared relieved to see the music therapist. She spoke softly about her husband, expressing a feeling of powerlessness, of not knowing what to do for him, as he could no longer ask her to do anything. The music therapist suggested she choose a song for the therapist to sing that might be meaningful to the patient. She selected a song the patient had chosen many times before, and the therapist began to sing, inviting the wife to join in if she desired. Quietly, almost inaudibly, the wife began to sing along. The music therapist asked her to choose a second song and, as she did, she shared its importance in their life's journey. The wife proceeded to choose more songs, telling their life's story and singing softly to her husband with the support of the music therapist. After songs she would touch his hand or say a few words to him, "Honey, remember when we …." This session provided a therapeutic intervention for the patient and his wife, movement toward relationship completion … and an opportunity for her to be the caregiver in a meaningful way. (p. 446)

Magee (1999) sings familiar precomposed songs with adults with multiple sclerosis. In a research study comparing the impact of singing familiar precomposed songs with improvising, she found that precomposed songs helped the patients connect to important people and events in their past with which the songs were associated. Her discussion includes many examples of the impact of these songs on the patients.

Considerations

Sing-alongs are sometimes misunderstood as being *all* that music therapists do. This is certainly not the case. Some music therapists even avoid sing-alongs because they don't want to fall into this stereotype. There are actually some very appropriate uses for sing-alongs. By using music from the client's life in the sing-along, the therapist gives the client something to which to relate. This may lead to a higher level of involvement than with many other approaches.

Keep the music that you will need on hand and be familiar enough with it so that you can accompany or assist *on the spot.* Music therapists have varying opinions on whether music needs to be memorized or whether it is satisfactory for the therapist to use the music as they play or sing. The best guidance is not to let your attention to the music compromise your attention to your clients. If this means that you must memorize music, by all means do so. It is always a good idea to have some familiar songs memorized so that you can be spontaneous when the need arises. You will also want to develop the ability to play, accompany, and sing using music or chord charts while giving most of your attention to your clients. In your beginning work, choose songs that are familiar to you, songs that you can accompany and sing while keeping your primary focus on the clients. You will naturally develop your repertoire of songs as you gain experience.

Materials

Some materials, including numerous books of music for instrumental activities, have been suggested in this chapter. These are all useful, and it is highly recommended that you be familiar with them. There are many other resources. If you are not able to find what you need in the available books, though, you may choose to compose your own music. After all, many of the pieces in the books mentioned in this chapter were inspired by people's clinical needs.

As with other art forms, there are guidelines for composing music to be used effectively in performing experiences. While extensive instruction in composing is beyond the scope of this book, we can point you to some good resources, including *Music for the Hearing-Impaired and Other Special Populations* by Robbins and Robbins (1980) and *Songwriting for Music Therapists* by Brunk (1997).

While the focus of some of these materials is on composing music *with* clients, much of what is written also applies to composing *for* clients. Briefly, you must be sure that the parts that you intend for clients to sing or play are appropriate for their needs and skills. In general, you will have better success with brief instrumental parts than with more complex ones (although there are certainly situations in which more complex parts may be useful). If you are going to be directing a group of clients, consider how many people will be able to play at once and how you will let them know who is to play; let these considerations guide your development of the musical content. When composing lyrics, be sure that they follow the inflection of speech and that the most important words fall on the strong beats. These are just a few very basic suggestions for composing; the books mentioned above have more extensive instructions.

You will need songbooks for many sing-alongs. Of course, the songs should be appropriate for the ages of the people in your sessions. For most purposes, having the words alone will suffice, but there will be situations in which you also will want to provide the music, either the melody alone or sometimes even the harmonization. It is often a good idea to have song sheets in a book with numbered pages and a table of contents to help people find the songs during the sessions. Some songbooks are commercially available, and you can also make your own. Two good collections that include very old songs are *Sing Along, Senior Citizens* by Grant (1973) and *Come Join the Geri-Tones* (1980).

For clients with more complex physical disabilities, it may be more helpful to use single song sheets, which are easier to hold. This facilitates attention and is physically less demanding for weakened or deformed hands. You may also find situations in which laminating lyric sheets, providing clipboards, or the use of a music stand will be necessary to facilitate success.

Tips for Using

Many of the considerations mentioned under Materials apply to this section. As you use re-creative experiences in your sessions, you will be using many of the conducting and leadership skills that you have developed. Although your style will vary with the situation, some of the sessions that you lead using these strategies may seem as though they are for entertainment or for education. It is up to you as therapist and session facilitator to ensure that you are working toward therapeutic goals. In a sing-along, for instance, remember to pay attention to what your clients would like to sing, why they would like to sing it, how they sing, and their memories of and associations to the songs. All of these things make the session more therapeutic—although it may also be entertaining!

As another example, if you are leading a group that is playing simple instruments and using a color-coded chart, it might be easy to feel that you are conducting a recreational activity rather than a music therapy session. These types of experiences *do* have some things in common—you must conduct the group with skill in order for them to play at the correct time. But, as therapist, you want to do more than provide a successful musical experience. You want to be sure that each client is playing the instrument that is best for his or her needs and skills and that each person is doing as much of the playing as he or she can do—and you want to provide assistance when needed. You may also want the clients to talk about how they feel about their playing. These are what make the session go beyond a valuable musical experience to become music therapy.

Assignments—Re-creative Experiences

These assignments should help you to deepen your understanding of the use of re-creative experiences in music therapy:

- Describe a time when you observed a therapist using a re-creative experience (a videotape or demonstration is okay). Based on the re-creative experiences suggested by Bruscia (2014b) and described in the first two paragraphs of this chapter, are you able to identify the specific type of re-creative experience that was implemented? What did you observe in the responses of the client(s) that could help the therapist to determine if the experience was beneficial?
- Considering the goals and objectives you already have identified for your client(s), is a re-creative experience an appropriate intervention to help meet these goals? If so, what qualities of a re-creative experience make it beneficial? How could you structure the intervention to include a re-creative experience? Find an example in the music therapy literature, perhaps a case study, that supports your thoughts about this.

- If re-creative experiences are indicated by the goals and objectives set for your client(s), which type or types of re-creative experiences might be beneficial? How will you determine which type or types of re-creative experiences to include, based on the anticipated benefits? How can you best prepare yourself to organize, present, develop, and process the experience?
- Find two examples of the use of re-creative experiences with your current population in the literature; try to locate one example of use in individual therapy and another example of group work. Describe them and provide the sources.
- For the current client(s) you are observing and/or with whom you are working, ask your clinical supervisor to describe some possible applications of re-creative experiences that have been or could be implemented. If re-creative experiences have been used in previous sessions, how have the client(s) responded? If re-creative experiences have not been used, is there a reason that they are counterindicated? Or, does your supervisor think that there could be benefits in providing such an experience, and, if so, are you able to participate in the development and/or presentation of a re-creative experience?

10 Compositional Experiences

In compositional experiences, the therapist helps the client write songs, lyrics, or instrumental pieces or create any kind of musical product, including music videos or audio recordings. The therapist typically takes responsibility for the more technical aspects of this process. Goals addressed may include skill development in the areas of decision-making; creating structures and organizing thoughts, materials, and content to work within the structures; developing strategies so that others can re-create the structures; and synthesizing parts into wholes (Bruscia, 2014b).

Variations include: *song transformation,* where the client changes only a part of an existing song while maintaining the balance of the original song; *songwriting,* where the client composes an original song or part of it (lyrics, melody, etc.) with help from the therapist and the song is written down or recorded; *instrumental composition,* which is similar to songwriting but for one or more instruments; *notational activities,* where the client creates a notational system and then composes a piece using it or provides notation for a precomposed piece; and *music collages,* in which the client selects and sequences sounds, songs, and words to produce a recording that explores autobiographical or therapeutic issues (Bruscia, 2014b).

Baker (2015), who has broad experience and has conducted extensive research on songwriting, suggests that methods of songwriting can be divided into three types: (a) methods that emphasize lyric creation, which includes fill-in-the-blank and song parody techniques (Baker labels as "song parody" techniques what Bruscia (2014b) calls "song transformation;" the authors will use Bruscia's term when referring to these techniques); (b) methods that emphasize both lyric and music creation, which includes rapping or singing over original music and song collages; and (c) methods that emphasize music creation, which include mash-ups (blending together the recordings of two or more prerecorded songs to form a new work), pastiche (the songwriter imitates or borrows motifs, techniques, or forms from one or more sources), hodgepodge (a form of pastiche that combines seemingly incongruent motifs, styles, and forms), and original songwriting within known structures. Two books that are very useful for learning songwriting techniques are Baker and Wigram (2005) and Baker (2015). A variety of perspectives on the use of rap and hip-hop are provided in *Therapeutic Uses of Rap and Hip-Hop* by Hadley and Yancy (2012).

Children with Special Needs

Composition experiences with children with special needs often concentrate on providing the client with an opportunity to assert some control over the way in which he or she obtains, retains, and retrieves a broad range of educational and developmental skills and knowledge, particularly in academic and social settings. Song transformation as well as songwriting can be productive experiences for these children. Eliciting information from the child about concepts that hold importance in life (e.g., family, friends, teachers, classroom rules) and that impact academic achievement can be an empowering experience as well as a learning tool. While extensive guidance and support from the therapist would be needed, engaging children in music collages could be very exciting and rewarding with the resulting tangible outcome of their own music video.

Adolescents and Adults with Intellectual and Developmental Disabilities

Because there is such a range of cognitive and language function in adults with developmental disabilities, composition experiences may take many different forms and functions in therapy. Song transformation is often a way to provide a client with first-time success, as the use of a song that is already familiar to the client alleviates concerns about creating melody, harmonic structure, and so forth. Often, lyric creation in the context of a familiar song structure (whether as part of song transformation or as a step toward creating an entirely original composition) may serve as a safe avenue for emotional expression. In some instances, simply engaging a client or group in conversation that is topic-specific and notating their responses can furnish enough information to create lyrics for a song. The therapist may need to establish the topic initially and facilitate the conversation, making certain that the subject matter is important to the clients. Compositional experiences can be used to support clients with a broad range of goals, including coming to closure with a therapist, developing a tool for retrieving sequences of information, and recognizing important accomplishments.

Adults with Psychiatric Disorders

Many clients in treatment for psychiatric disorders are encouraged to express themselves verbally. Music therapy offers the opportunity to channel that expression into nonverbal forms. Creating song melodies that express a specific mood or idea can be done with individuals or in small groups. Clients may wish to add words or may prefer to complete the experience with musical sound alone.

When creating lyrics with these clients, the lyric experience may be used as a tool for expressing a specific idea or mood (here is what is on my mind), as a means of looking at a topic or problem (this is what I think/feel about ____), as a tool for problem-solving (when I think/feel ____, I begin to wonder ____ and then I ____), or as a medium for telling a story (before I ____, but now I ____; someday I hope to ____). Clients often begin this experience by stating, "I don't know how to write a song." The therapist's role is to guide the client through the process, offering the level of structure needed to achieve success.

Another form of composing can be accomplished by inviting the clients to create lyrics about a topic. The therapist then improvises music to express the emotional message of the lyrics, accepting guidance from the client as to how to shape the improvisation. Clients have responded to this style of composing with such statements as, "That music sounds like I feel. It makes me feel that others can understand me."

More structured compositional experiences can be designed in which clients create a melody using a predetermined pattern or code, such as when implementing notational activities described earlier in this chapter. Clients can create a short motif or a longer phrase of music that can be joined together to create a composition. This can be done in a group setting or with an individual client.

Older Adults with Age-Related Needs

Older adults may have varying levels of cognitive functioning. At most levels, they can be engaged in songwriting or compositional experiences with varying amounts of structure. For those with cognitive impairments, the goals are likely to focus on giving expression to thoughts and feelings in a form that is easier than expressing them verbally. The degree of structure and the therapist's facilitation skill will be the keys to success for those with cognitive impairments. For those with higher levels of cognitive functioning, goals may focus more on expression of emotion.

Group composition also meets goals related to working together, feeling part of a group, and achieving a sense of accomplishment. For example, a group may be guided through a thematic discussion at a very simple level (such as "Name something you think about in the spring"). A list of personal ideas may be gathered together and orchestrated with sound or may be given a melody and even a harmonic structure (perhaps chosen from two selections played for the group). Those with cognitive impairments can often make choices between two options; thus, in composing experiences at this level, the therapist must provide much of the material from which the group will work if members are unable to spontaneously offer ideas.

People in Medical Settings

Hospitalization is filled with uncertainty. Creation of song lyrics or melodies and harmonies provides patients with a structure to express the emotions behind their fears and concerns. These songs often look at the realities of the hospital experience and project into the future the patient's wishes and hopes. The therapist helps the patient to structure the expression and to process its meaning when appropriate. The therapist's skill in facilitating the composition influences the patient's response, especially for patients with no previous musical training or experience. The therapist might offer the beginning of a lyrical or melodic line and invite the patient to complete the phrase. The therapist might brainstorm with the patient about the hospital experience, identify themes, and assist the patient in creating phrases that correspond to those themes. Music might then be created based on the patient's choices. When patients are asked to choose the tempo, mode, harmonic patterns, direction of the melody, and other elements of the music, this greatly assists them in composing music that reflects their inner self.

Songwriting can also serve as an evaluative tool for illuminating progress in a rehabilitation setting. For example, when utilized with those who have had traumatic brain injuries or strokes, the complexity and lucidity of the lyrics, in combination with harmonic, rhythmic, and melodic sophistication, can provide the therapist with tangible outcomes for measuring improvements in emotional stability and long-term recall as well as offer a window into the client's outlook for the future.

Uses in the Music Therapy Literature

Children with Special Needs

Songwriting with very young children frequently takes place through improvisation, since they do not have the reading skills required for actual songwriting. Therefore, the examples of the use of this technique in the music therapy literature are often with older children and adolescents, although there are also some examples of composition experiences being used with younger children. Roberts and McFerran (2013) undertook a mixed methods content analysis of lyrics written by young, bereaved children (ages 7–12 years) who were participating in individual music therapy. The researchers sought to determine if the children were able to use songwriting effectively to address their grief. A total of 49 songs were created, 18 of which were exclusively devoted to grief. Other songs focused on the emotions that resulted from grief (e.g., sadness, anger, guilt, feelings of injustice and abandonment), while still others contained more peaceful content (e.g., happiness that the lost loved one is no longer suffering) and various sorts of psychological and spiritual experiences.

Gfeller (1987) used songwriting as a tool for reading and language remediation as part of the language experience approach, which utilizes children's spoken language as a basis for writing and then reading. She describes a sequence of steps for using songwriting to elicit these language experience stories.

Rio and Tenney (2002) describe the use of composition in a case study of a 16-year-old male in a juvenile offenders' residence. After the therapist had a sense of what the boy wanted to write about and the style, the boy was given a sheet of paper with some original lyrics of a song and then blanks in which he could complete the lines. He wrote several songs in this way, one of which contained numerous expletives. Later, when his attitude had changed, he altered the song to reflect a more positive attitude.

Robb (1996) describes a number of songwriting techniques for helping adolescents who have had traumatic injuries to restore emotional and physical well-being. She includes a fill-in-the-blank format, group songwriting, improvisational songwriting, and discharge songs. Her article offers additional suggestions for developing songwriting techniques.

Adolescents and Adults with Intellectual and Developmental Disabilities

Although the use of composing with people with developmental disabilities needs to be at a very basic level due to limitations in language and other skills, Boxill (1985) illustrates its use with this population. Using call-and-response singing, group members called out foods that they would eat on Thanksgiving Day, and each was put into a verse of a Thanksgiving song (p. 152). Fischer (1991) describes her work with a young adult male who had developmental disabilities and autism. Through a combination of discussion and drawing, the client was able to engage and participate in songwriting experiences that started with safe topics such as food, resulting in the "Food Song" and progressing to more challenging subjects that produced the "Fear Song" and the "Self Song" (pp. 359–371).

In discussing songwriting with a group of adolescents with moderate intellectual disabilities, McFerran (2010) describes similar procedures in that the therapist must play an active and somewhat directive role in facilitating a positive outcome. In the scenario provided, the six 14-year-old group members are all enthusiastic about the prospect of writing a song but are unable to agree on a topic, each calling out different ideas such as sports, dancing, going to the movies, etc. Accepting and valuing all contributions, the therapist discerns a common thread: things the group members enjoy doing with family and friends. The next challenge is agreeing on style, with some members preferring rap over singing. All are able to accept a structure that incorporates both styles. The finished product successfully incorporated each individual member's interests and musical preferences.

"Jazzy" (a pseudonym for an adolescent with learning and attention issues as well as related behavioral challenges) worked with Polen and Hunter individually over the course of two school placements ("Jazzy," Polen, & Hunter, 1999). He described the value of music therapy experiences in his overall development, particularly as related to emotional expression, self-esteem, and academic achievement, indicating that the processes of moving from shared improvisation to compositional experiences, which included notation, recording, and playback, were the most meaningful and pleasurable aspects of his therapy. The enduring products resulting from the compositional experiences also allowed for him to share his journey with others.

Adults with Psychiatric Disorders

Eyre (2013) identifies songwriting as a frequently used intervention for patients in psychiatric treatment, especially in group work. She describes variations of this experience that are useful for short-term inpatient treatment, suggesting that the amount of structure in the experience can be altered to meet the needs of the group. The simplest form of songwriting involves substitution of words to make a song more personally meaningful. Creating song parodies (keeping the existing music but creating new lyrics) may result from a discussion among the clients or brainstorming a list of words associated with a topic. The music therapist assists the clients in creating phrases that become the lyrics for the song parody. A more challenging form of songwriting involves the creation of new lyrics and new music. It is suggested that using a specific genre may provide structure to this approach.

Cassity and Cassity (2006) suggest several methods of song composition that may be used in working with adults with psychiatric disorders. They focus the work by saying (p. 136), "The goal is to get a tangible 'black and white' copy of the patient's true feelings. Does the patient write lyrics that reflect appropriate self-awareness, emotions, and contact with the environment? Does the patient give suggestions for lyrics based on her own thoughts and feelings?" Their suggestions include: Give each client a work sheet and ask each to contribute to the parody, using a familiar melody; have each client make up a lyrical verse to the melody of a familiar song; have each client create one line of lyrics; use blues form to involve clients in writing lyrics, beginning with the music therapist singing lyrics that are already written (with accompaniment), then prompting the client to try new lyrics; assist the client in deciding upon a melody and chord progression that best expresses lyrics that are reflective of the client's feelings; help the client to hum an unknown melody, then compose lyrics to the melody; and have the client fill in words that have been deleted from a song.

McFerran (2010) provides an example of the use of lyric substitution with a group of adolescents in an inpatient psychiatric setting. The group initially selected a song that would serve as the basis for their work by voting on several choices. The therapist was fairly directive, suggesting that they change the words to include examples of coping strategies that they used when they were feeling down. This led to a number of contributions and some discussion of these strategies. The task for the reported session was to come up with lyrics, with plans for the following session to focus on accompaniment with instruments.

Gallagher and Steele (2002) describe a music therapy program for people with combined substance abuse and mental illness issues. They find songwriting to be a particular favorite of the clients. They share their use of several songwriting techniques and give examples of the resulting songs.

Rolvsjord (2010) describes individual therapy over the course of a couple of years with a woman with mental health challenges. Songwriting was a major component of the therapy, with many of the lyrics beginning as poems written by the client during her numerous periods of hospitalization for psychotic episodes during which she also engaged in self-harm. Many of the early poems had childhood trauma and her resulting anger as their theme. As therapy progressed, the content of the poems did as well, with focus areas transitioning to those of recovery, independence, emerging strength, and struggles with self-confidence. The client was able to report on her experience, sharing insights with her therapist regarding the opportunities for communication and coping strategies that the process of songwriting provided.

Older Adults with Age-Related Needs

Although composing and songwriting are not widely used with people with dementia, there are examples of their use. Chavin (1991) uses lyric substitution and an adaptation of that technique, silly/nonsensical songs. Silly/nonsensical songs are composed by deleting words from a familiar song and then asking participants to give different kinds of words, "the more unusual, the better" (p. 66). Chavin instructs, "After the list is finished, fill in the words on a large piece of paper for everyone to read and sing the 'silly song' you've just written" (p. 66).

Silber and Hes (1995) speak of their work using songwriting with patients diagnosed with Alzheimer's disease. Although they acknowledge the apparent contradiction in having people with Alzheimer's disease write songs, since songwriting ability seems dependent upon skills that people with Alzheimer's have lost, they report that clients were able to write songs and poetry with the proper assistance. They describe three techniques for achieving this: (a) The music therapist sings one phrase at a time from an existing melody and encourages the clients to find and adapt words to it, (b) the music therapist composes a new melody and the clients provide a text, and (c) the music therapist provides a theme for writing poetry to background music. The authors provide examples of songs written in their sessions.

Hong and Choi (2011) did a study of the effects of songwriting-oriented activities on the cognitive abilities of 30 older adults, most of whom had Alzheimer's disease. Their experimental group participated in the songwriting activities, while the control group had standard treatment. The main stage of songwriting involved asking participants to tell their past experiences related to various cognitive functions and fill in the blanks of songs with the contents discussed or replace existing lyrics with content related to cognitive functions, then improvise songs as well as rhythms. The final stage reinforced songwriting through activities such as singing the songs that were written, singing with instruments or with movements, or playing games with the songs. They assessed the cognitive functions of the participants using the Mini-Mental Status Examination (MMSE-K) and found a number of positive changes in cognitive functioning among those who participated in the songwriting.

Using songwriting with retirees who exhibited no cognitive deterioration, Baker and Ballantyne (2013) conducted five sessions, one using song transformation and the next four using Baker's (2005) model of therapeutic songwriting, in which the group leaders facilitated participants' brainstorming, then organized their thoughts and identified core ideas or feelings, then created the song. Following the five sessions, the retirees and leaders formed a choir and sang the song to others. They found that the program "stimulated their enjoyment, positively affected emotions, and improved well-being. They experienced enhanced connection with each other and with others in the broader community. They experienced a sense of accomplishment, meaning, and engagement in creating and performing their own songs" (p. 7).

People in Medical Settings

Hadley (1996) expresses the value of using songs with children in the hospital:

> Songs may be selected by the therapist to give reassurance, to deal with separation anxiety and isolation by offering comforting images of home and family, to stimulate expression of feelings, and to instill hope about recovery. Alternatively, children may create their own songs. The songwriting process can enhance a child's expression of feelings. (p. 20)

Whitehead-Pleaux and Spall (2014) present a number of uses of technology in working with children with burn injuries. Many of these facilitate song composition. They describe the use of GarageBand to help two girls cope with their anxiety about their upcoming surgeries. They wrote the lyrics together, each sharing their feelings as part of the song. The therapist then assisted them in composing the music by creating loops on GarageBand. They agreed on drum loops, then on additional instruments. They then recorded the words. At a later time, the therapist brought them a copy of the lyrics and a CD with their song on it. This composition helped them to share their concerns about the surgeries and relate to someone else who shared the same concerns.

Silverman (2012) examined the effectiveness of a single group songwriting session as an intervention with patients in a detoxification unit. He found that patients who participated in a single music therapy session experienced significant improvements in their motivation and readiness for treatment when compared with patients who did not participate in music therapy. Borling (2011) also uses songwriting with people in recovery from addiction. He provides the following sequence: Clients are asked to sing a verse that has been composed by the music therapist, followed by the creation of the patients' own verses using a structure that allows their lyrics to fit musically. He says that "the final challenge of this exercise is to sing one's original verse for the group, accompanied by guitar (or piano)" (p. 343).

M. Murphy (1983) provides a summary of the use of songwriting with substance abuse clients in a group setting. During twice-weekly sessions that alternate between one focused on improvisation and one on songwriting, the group collaborates on developing lyrics and then works to determine the accompanying music. The focus is to help group members gain insight into their addictions and actively participate in treatment.

O'Brien (2006) created an opera with cancer patients and professional singers. She found overall themes of anger, fear, humor, suffering, and peace, leading her to conclude that creating the opera was a transformative experience for the participants.

O'Callaghan (2005) discusses songs written by palliative care patients in music therapy. Her steps include: brainstorm on a selected theme, organize ideas into related themes, offer music elements, and provide title–transcribe into manuscript–record. She emphasizes that these are flexible steps and, of course, that the needs of the patient must be met by whatever procedures are followed.

Reuer (2005) developed a *Music Therapy Toolbox* for medical settings. One of the items in this toolbox is lyric substitution. She includes specific songs that she has found successful and suggestions for what can be substituted in them.

Shultis and Gallagher (2015) offer an example of helping a patient create original lyrics and melody. The patient described his stressors and from that discussion was able to find statements to reflect his feelings about his circumstances. The music therapist helped him to fit his ideas into melodic phrases that fit the 12-bar blues pattern he had chosen from options offered by the music therapist. The end product included possible coping strategies to help him withstand the needed medical care.

Considerations

There are many ways to structure composition, ranging from utilizing music and words from a precomposed song to substituting only single words, to helping the client compose a complete piece of music. These techniques provide opportunities to address the needs of clients on various levels. Several articles and books in the literature provide guidelines for composition (e.g., Brunk, 1997; Pattison, 1991; Schmidt, 1983).

Different compositional techniques require different levels of skill from the music therapist. It is recommended that you begin with techniques that are within your skill level and become comfortable using them, then gradually attempt those that require more skill.

Materials

If you are simply composing a piece of music, you will need a way to notate and/or record the composition. If you are working with a group, the writing should be large enough for all to see to enable them to participate in the process. Consider recording the composition for later transcription and development and bringing it to the next session in a more polished form.

Many electronic music technologies (EMTs) that can facilitate compositional experiences are available. *Music Technology in Therapeutic and Health Settings,* edited by Magee (2014), is an invaluable resource for clinical uses of EMTs and other uses of music technology.

Other techniques require some materials. If you are using song transformation, in which the client is changing part of the song, you may want to have the words, melody, or harmony of the original song written down for reference. If you want to write down or record the song that results from the experience, you will need a pencil and paper or audio recorder. If you are doing instrumental composition, you will want to have the instruments for which you are composing. If you are doing a notational activity, you will need paper on which to write the notational system. If you are making a music collage, you will need to have a collection of songs from which to select the portions to record. These will generally be recorded music but could also be performed live. You will also need a means of recording the collage.

Tips for Using

Composing music can be very intimidating for students and professionals, since you do not know how the composition is going to end! Many music therapy students and therapists do not have the skills to make up accompaniments spontaneously and thus are afraid to attempt compositions. One suggestion for dealing with this is to begin with simple techniques and then build up to more complicated techniques. Another suggestion is to just do it! It is often more frightening to think about composing than to actually do it.

It is likely that a lot of the fear involved in composing comes from feeling that you are trying to create something out of nothing, and the accompanying sense of inadequacy. In a manner of speaking, this is true. However, when composing for the clinical setting, you already have lots of materials available to you. You just have to know where to look—and listen—for them.

Songs and instrumental pieces are created all the time in the course of a therapy session. If you are able to audio- or videotape your sessions (make sure that you have permission and that any required confidentiality forms are processed), this can be quite helpful not only in reviewing client behaviors and your own interactions with clients, but also in remembering and transcribing important events. These significant events may take many forms, including verbal, vocal, or lyrical and rhythmic, harmonic, melodic, or timbral. Melodic or rhythmic themes that escaped you when you were in the midst of facilitating the session may suddenly emerge when reviewing session tapes. Even if the tape review doesn't result in a set of lyrics, a melody, or an instrumental piece, it will most certainly help you to sharpen your ability to recognize and identify patterns, musical and otherwise, in your work.

While it is true that many songs and other compositions used in therapy are spontaneously born in a music therapy session, there are other times when a music therapist must compose a piece outside of therapy and bring that composition into the session for the benefit of clients. As mentioned earlier, start with simple techniques and always keep in mind the clients for whom you are composing in order to ensure that the piece will provide them with a musically and therapeutically successful experience. If the composition is meaningful and motivating, it will encourage participation and success and may endure as a useful tool for other clients as well.

Care must be taken when considering whether melodic material should have words or be instrumental. The lyric line must follow the natural rhythm and intonation of the spoken word in order to fully support and elicit the verbal or vocal response from the client. You may find that chanting the lyrics while tapping a basic pulse will help you to determine the melodic rhythm. This naturally leads you to determine where the accents are and thus drives the melodic direction. With regard to the lyrics themselves, you may obtain them from the clients during earlier sessions or you may develop them yourself, perhaps to impart information to the clients within a song structure.

If you are working on a melodic line for instrumental use, think carefully about the skills of the client who might play the melody and then write a part for a specific instrument. Is he or she able to play just one tone bar, play two in sequence, or use a full xylophone? Perhaps you are writing a keyboard part. Will the client use one or two hands? How much digital (finger) control does he or she have?

Another way to begin to gain the skills for using composing in music therapy sessions is to listen to examples of the music that you expect to compose. Listening to the blues or rap, for instance, may help your compositions to more easily emerge in the desired musical style and *feel.*

There are, of course, many other considerations when composing music for therapy. The ideas in this chapter can help to get you started.

Assignments—Compositional Experiences

These assignments can help to deepen your understanding of the use of the compositional experiences covered in this chapter:

- Describe a time when you observed a therapist using a compositional experience (a videotape or demonstration is okay). Based on the compositional experiences suggested by Bruscia (2014b) and described in the first two paragraphs of this chapter, are you able to identify the specific type of compositional experience that was implemented? What did you observe in the responses of the client(s) that could help the therapist to determine if the experience was beneficial?
- Think about incorporating the use of a compositional experience in one of your sessions. Considering the goals and objectives you already have identified for your client(s), how could you structure the intervention to include a compositional experience? Is a compositional experience appropriate for addressing the goals and objectives identified? If so, which type or types of compositional experiences might be beneficial for your client(s)? How will you determine which type or types of compositional experiences to include, based on the anticipated benefits? How can you best prepare yourself to organize, present, develop, and process the experience?
- Find two examples of the use of compositional experiences with your current

population in the literature; try to locate one example of use in individual therapy and another example of group work. Describe them and provide the sources.

- For the current client(s) you are observing and/or with whom you are working, ask your clinical supervisor to describe some possible applications of compositional experiences that have been or could be implemented. If compositional experiences have been used in previous sessions, how have the client(s) responded? If compositional experiences have not been used, is there a reason that they are contraindicated? Or, does your supervisor think that there could be benefits in providing such an experience? If so, are you able to participate in the development and/or presentation of a compositional experience?

11 | Receptive Experiences

In receptive experiences, the client listens to music and responds silently, verbally, or in another modality. The music may be of any genre and in any form, that is, recorded or live. The music is selected and presented in a manner that targets the therapeutic goals of the client. Goal areas may include those of physical, emotional, intellectual, aesthetic, or spiritual focus. Music therapy utilizing listening experiences may also be referred to as *receptive music therapy* (Bruscia, 2014b).

There are many variations of receptive experiences, including *somatic listening,* where vibrations, sounds, and music directly influence the client's body; *music for pain management,* where music is used to help reduce the effects of pain; *music relaxation or meditative listening,* where music is used to help with relaxation, meditation, or stimulation of the senses; *subliminal listening,* where sounds or music are used to mask the delivery of subliminal messages to the unconscious mind; *stimulative listening,* to stimulate the senses, bring alertness, or elevate mood; *eurhythmic listening,* where music is used to rhythmically organize and monitor the client's motor behaviors; *perceptual listening,* where music listening is used to improve various auditory skills; *action listening,* where musical cues are used to elicit specific behavioral responses; *contingent listening,* where listening serves as a reward for a particular response; *mediational listening,* where music is paired with information or experiences to help in learning or to make something more memorable and retrievable; *music appreciation activities,* where music is used to help the client understand various components and functions of music; *song (music) reminiscence,* where music listening evokes memories of past experiences; *song (music) regression,* where music is used to help the client re-experience the past; *induced song (music) recall,* where the therapist helps the client to recall, either consciously or unconsciously, a song that spontaneously comes into the client's awareness; *song (music) communication,* where the therapist asks the client to bring in a piece of music that communicates something; *song (lyric) discussion,* where the therapist brings in a song to serve as a stimulus for discussion; *projective listening,* where the therapist presents music for the client to identify, describe, interpret, or free-associate to; *imaginal listening,* which serves to evoke and support imaginal thinking or inner processes, often while in an altered state of consciousness; *and self-listening,* where the client listens to a recording of their own musicing for the purpose of reflection (Bruscia, 2014b).

In addition to references included in this chapter, there are many good sources of information on receptive uses of music in therapy. A number of these are about Guided Imagery and Music and include *Music Consciousness: The Evolution of Guided Imagery and Music* by Bonny (2002); *Guided Imagery and Music: The Bonny Method and Beyond*, edited by Bruscia and Grocke (2002); and *Guided Imagery and Music in the Institutional Setting* by Summer (1990). In addition, the *Journal of the Association for Music and Imagery* contains many articles on Guided Imagery and Music. Hurt-Thaut and Johnson (2015) describe a number of Neurologic Music Therapy techniques, some of which are examples of receptive music therapy.

Children with Special Needs

Children are typically directed to *do* something as part of many listening experiences, as doing is a way of promoting children's involvement with the music. Thus, purely receptive experiences with children are somewhat limited. At times, the music therapist will use imagery and music with children, perhaps to help them think through a situation. Relaxation exercises appropriate to a child's level of functioning might be used and could include background music. The Somatron®, a device that produces physical vibrations when connected to a sound source and often used with guided imagery, can assist children's relaxation or sensory awareness.

Adolescents and Adults with Intellectual and Developmental Disabilities

The use of receptive experiences in therapy with adolescents and adults with intellectual and developmental disabilities (IDD) can be challenging, as often these clients do not possess the cognitive and attentional abilities to benefit from these experiences. Somatic listening, particularly through the use of vibroacoustic experiences such as can be presented through use of the Somatron®, is one area that can provide some clients with a tangible, externalized experience of relaxation. Many adolescents and adults with IDD may additionally suffer from emotional or behavioral difficulties. Vibroacoustic music experiences, paired with modeling and prompting from the music therapist, can help the person begin to learn new ways of processing and responding to external stimuli. Stimulative listening can support those individuals who may need arousal; this may be further enhanced by engaging such clients in eurhythmic listening and/or action listening. Contingent listening strategies may also prove beneficial for certain individuals.

Adults with Psychiatric Disorders

Listening to music is often the first step for adults with psychiatric disorders in becoming involved in the music therapy process. Music therapy may be unfamiliar to these clients, and the idea of playing instruments or singing may be uncomfortable or unappealing. Beginning with preferred music listening allows the therapist to build a relationship with clients based on a musical experience. Sharing preferred music (or music chosen from a selection of available recordings) with a group can be structured to allow clients to introduce themselves to the group, to tell something about themselves, or to present music that has meaning for them that they are not ready to share verbally. These clients also often appreciate the structured relaxation session with music, which lets them be the passive recipients of care instead of having to actively work at therapy. Listening to specific pieces of music or songs may also be used as a bridge to discussions of topics that are relevant to them. Monitoring their responses to a piece of music can be enlightening, as clients often develop increased self-awareness through receptive experiences.

Older Adults with Age-Related Needs

Reminiscence experiences offer several distinct benefits when working with older adults. First, for people nearing the end of their lives, accessing memories of their past can help them to validate the meaning of their lives. Second, when memory loss occurs, whether through normal aging or a more serious affliction such as Alzheimer's, past memories can often be more successfully accessed through reminiscence experiences. In addition, music appreciation sessions are often used to help maintain and stimulate the cognitive skills of well-functioning older adults.

Several variations of music listening can be used in working with older adults whose functioning has decreased markedly. The organization of motor behaviors that can be accomplished with eurhythmic listening can be very useful for people with decreased motor functioning, who may not respond as well to verbal commands as they do to music. Stimulative listening is often effective in helping to arouse and alert an individual, as well as providing support with reality orientation and contact with their environment and others in it. In addition, perceptual listening may help the auditory skills of people at lower levels of functioning.

Several other listening techniques lend themselves well to working with older adults. Somatic listening and music for pain management can both be used to stimulate or to decrease physical pain, for example. Music relaxation and meditative listening may both be used to help people relax and reduce stress.

People in Medical Settings

The focus of a hospitalization is the patient's physical recovery, and often little or no attention is given to the emotional impact of the hospitalization experience. Patients can find themselves experiencing emotions yet be unable to focus on them, describe them, or appreciate how they are connected to the hospitalization. When patients are offered or are able to choose music that expresses their emotional states, it can be a powerful acknowledgement of their internal experiences. This essentially nonverbal technique for clarifying emotional responses to hospitalization is also useful for patients on ventilators who are unable to talk.

Listening to music for relaxation and pain management is obviously very useful for medical patients. Patients may be assisted in choosing music to keep at bedside when they need to decrease anxiety, to induce sleep, or to manage pain. Listening may be coupled with imagery experiences to develop associational cues for relaxation or decreased pain. The development of associational cues is an adaptation of a technique used by Dolan (1991) for treating patients experiencing posttraumatic stress disorder resulting from sexual abuse. The client is asked to associate an image with a music-induced relaxation response. The client is then instructed to practice with this music and image until the image alone can evoke the relaxation response.

Uses in the Music Therapy Literature
Children with Special Needs

Although the majority of music therapy techniques for children involve them in making music, there are some examples of using music listening or background music with children. One of these is Herman's (1991) use of music as a background for playing with water, playing in sand, and finger painting with a 9-year-old boy with severe emotional difficulties. In each case, the music helped to structure the boy's work with these other media and thus contributed to the success of the treatment.

The use of vibroacoustic therapy with a 14-year-old boy with a moderate IDD and visual and motor disabilities was described by Persoons and De Backer (1997). The boy received vibroacoustic therapy prior to a music therapy session in which he played and improvised. After a number of sessions, it was found that his tension decreased markedly with the vibroacoustic therapy.

Wyatt (2002) gives several examples of the use of receptive music therapy techniques with juvenile offenders. One technique is "Name That Jam," in which the therapist records song samples that represent a variety of musical genres. The group is divided into teams, and clients work in groups to identify the artists and song titles. The goals are to provide a positive listening experience and to establish relationships, so interaction and cooperation are emphasized.

Katagiri (2009) used background music (improvised music reflective of emotions paired with verbal instruction) as a tool for developing emotional understanding in children with autism, finding it to be more effective than singing specially composed songs about emotions. Background music (45 minutes of classical adagios and Enya with tempos starting at 78 beats per minute and gradually dropping to 48 beats per minute) played at naptime and bedtime was also effective in improving the sleep quality of elementary school–age children when used for 3 weeks (Leepeng, 2004).

Adolescents and Adults with Intellectual and Developmental Disabilities

Boxill (1985) describes the use of receptive music therapy techniques in a group session with a 20-year-old woman with severe intellectual disabilities (pp. 127–131). When the woman's behavior became agitated, the therapist played a lullaby in an attempt to relax her, while the aide was instructed to take the woman's hands and sway back and forth with her, humming along with the therapist. While the woman moved to the music, she also began to hum, the first sounds that she had ever made in response to music. This led to the entire group's involvement in the humming and swaying and later to enough improvement in the woman's behavior that she was able to discontinue individual music therapy sessions in favor of group sessions. While swaying to music is an example of the use of listening experiences, or receptive music therapy, the humming would probably be considered a basic example of improvising or re-creating. This, then, is an example of how music experiences do not always occur in discrete categories but may cross over and include several at the same time.

While live music can be used as reinforcement, recorded music can also work in many situations; for example, in a study by Wolfe (1980), appropriate head posturing by individuals with cerebral palsy automatically triggered contingent music.

Grocke and Wigram (2007) describe the use of recorded music with individuals with intellectual disabilities, specifically indicating its use for outcomes such as improving attention or promoting relaxation. They suggest the value of receptive experiences in both individual and group work and how the planned use of recorded music can provide a natural break in the more active work of a music therapy session.

Adults with Psychiatric Disorders

Borczon (1997) describes listening to music, reading the lyrics, and discussing what has been heard with a group of adults in a chemical dependency recovery program. Group members guess what stage of treatment the singer might be in, which draws them into the music and helps them to reflect their own treatment issues. McFerran (2010) discusses the use of lyric analysis (song discussion) with a 16-year-old inpatient being treated for first episode psychosis. The goals for therapy include using music-elicited associations to generate memories, encouraging verbal processing, and promoting emotional expression. In the first session, the client is given responsibility for the song selection. Following quiet reflection, the therapist initiates the discussion before moving on to a second song selection. In this initial session, the implementation of song (music) reminiscence and song (lyric) discussion allowed the therapist to establish rapport with the client, providing a foundation for their working relationship and motivation for the client to return for follow-up sessions.

In her program for offenders with mental disorders, Reed (2002) created two music listening groups, soul and rock, based on client taste. Members of these groups chose recordings in advance and then played two selections of music during the session. Goals were to improve active listening skills, increase tolerance for group activity, increase tolerance of the choices of others, and develop constructive use of leisure time.

Eyre (2011a) employed several receptive music therapy techniques in her work with Julie, a young woman who was diagnosed with psychosis and had experienced multiple traumas. In the early stages of their work, Julie did not speak, so Eyre used songs that Julie's mother reported her to like. These helped her make contact with Julie. Later, Julie was able to choose her own music. Eyre also used listening experiences such as vocal improvisation with accompaniment to match Julie's mood, singing songs to access soothing feelings and encourage awareness of herself and others.

It is common for clients with psychiatric challenges to have difficulty talking about emotional states. Listening may lead to discussion of emotions and then to increased use of verbal descriptors to name and express emotion. As group members listen to and describe the music, they learn vocabulary for emotional expression from one another (Shultis, 1999).

Older Adults with Age-Related Needs

Several writers have described the use of listening to music in working with people with dementia. Ridder (Ridder & Wheeler, 2015) describes how singing to a woman who was in a state of panic helped to calm her down. Then, as she listened to songs sung by Plàcido Domingo, she would close her eyes, lean back in her chair, and sigh with relief. Also working with a woman with dementia, Van Bruggen-Rufi (Van Bruggen-Rufi & Vink, 2011) played the ukulele and sang music from a woman's Indonesian culture for a woman with dementia who felt alienated from others in her nursing facility. The authors felt that this helped the woman to connect to her memories and feel better.

Music listening has been used to stimulate reminiscence in older adults. Chavin (1991) and Cordrey (1994) describe the use of reminiscence groups with people with dementia, both making the point that reminiscence activities can help to stimulate memories that those with dementia may not be able to retrieve on their own. These authors include topics around which to focus the reminiscence, including "You Must Have Been a Beautiful Baby," suggested by Chavin (pp. 44–45) and including various aspects of babies, including discussion of memories of being pregnant and having babies. Other songs and themes suggested by Chavin include "Toyland," "School Days," and "Sentimental Journey." Chavin reminds us that the memories are not always positive, saying that "tearful reactions to music and memories are not uncommon and are not always negative" (p. 42). Cordrey suggests topics such as "Memories of Dad," "Symbols of Christmas," and "School Days." Shaw (1993) provides a number of examples of the use of reminiscence with older adults, oriented around seasonal themes presented for each month of the year.

Vibroacoustic therapy shows promising results with people who have Alzheimer's disease. In a study that assessed the effect of stimulating their somatosensory system using 40 Hz sound stimulation versus visual stimulation using DVDs, the sound stimulation had a greater effect on mental status, observed emotions, and behavioral observations than did the DVDs (Clements-Cortes et al., 2016).

Receptive music experiences are also used with older adults who do not have dementia. One type, such as music appreciation, may be especially helpful for those with higher cognitive abilities and may provide a useful source of stimulation. These discussions will often lead to the processing of personal issues (Bright, 1991) as well as reactions to the music. Other receptive experiences may be structured for people with different needs, such as a need for comfort or to help with orientation. Gfeller and Hanson (1995) provide examples of how to structure listening to music into sessions.

Listening experiences may also be used to reduce stress. Hanser (1990) and Hanser and Thompson (1994) utilized specially programmed tapes in a study of methods for reducing stress in older adults in their homes. Clair (1996) describes a number of receptive music techniques that can be useful in helping residents to relax and relieve stress and pain.

People in Medical Settings

There are many examples of the use of receptive techniques in medical settings. Included in this category are some instances of recorded music being used by medical personnel as an adjunct to medical treatments or situations, classified by Dileo (1999) as music medicine (see Standley, 2000, for additional information on these uses of music). The examples presented below, however, are of receptive music therapy techniques that are utilized by music therapists.

Music therapy in medical settings includes applications of music in a vibrational form. Skille (1997) reports the use of vibroacoustic therapy with applications in the areas of pain disorders, muscular conditions, pulmonary disorders, general physical ailments, and psychological disorders. Naghdi et al. (2015) found that patients with fibromyalgia who received low-frequency sound stimulation made significant improvements as measured on the Fibromyalgia Impact Questionnaire, Jenkins Sleep Scale, and Pain Disability Index, as well as in muscle motion and tone and self-report. The low-frequency vibrations can be presented through a number of forms, including the Somatron®. Numerous other examples of the use of vibroacoustic therapy (not all in medical settings) are provided by Wigram and Dileo (1997).

Reuer (2005) describes a number of techniques for utilizing music and imagery and music listening in medical settings. Meadows (2015) describes music and imagery practices for people who have cancer as being along a continuum of experiences loosely divided into three levels: (a) symptom management, (b) supportive music and imagery, and (c) reconstructive music and imagery. These are based on the level or depth at which the work occurs. Music and imagery interventions for specific medical conditions are described by Hertrampf and Klinken (2015) for women with cancer and Wärja and Klinken (2015) for women recovering from gynecological cancer.

Hurt, Rice, McIntosh, and Thaut (1998) utilized Rhythmic Auditory Stimulation (RAS), a technique of Neurologic Music Therapy, in gait training for patients with traumatic brain injury. This technique utilizes the organizing ability of rhythm to help patients with various gait problems to organize and coordinate their movements. The music therapist assesses the patient's current gait and selects music that will support the desired changes. There is extensive empirical evidence of the effectiveness of RAS (see https://nmtacademy.files.wordpress.com/2015/09/sensorimotorclinical.pdf).

Grocke and Wigram (2007) provide suggestions for the selection of music for infants and young children in hospital environments, outlining specific strategies for receptive music therapy experiences for hospitalized children for specific outcomes of relaxation, pain reduction, alleviation of fear and anxiety, distraction, respiratory integrity, imaginative thinking, and overall improvement of the experience during their hospitalization. They further describe receptive experiences for children with sleep difficulties related to mental health challenges in an inpatient setting; for children in palliative care; and for supports in classroom settings to address issues related to stress, self-management of behavior, challenges with concentration, creative thinking, and general pleasure. Finally, suggestions are also offered for parent use at home in assisting relaxation and sleep.

Nöcker-Ribaupierre, as cited in Frohne-Hagemann (2007), discusses the use of sound (live and recorded, and including the human voice) at the beginning of life, confirming that the only form of music therapy that premature infants can participate in is receptive music therapy. Whether the targeted outcomes are those of a medical music therapy model, relationship-oriented work, or providing a more normalized environment (and one in which the mother and/or father are included), the use of receptive methods can be crucial in supporting the development of these young and fragile clients.

Considerations

Receptive experiences come in many varieties. Some, such as music appreciation, are similar to what may be done in music education. Receptive experiences will be most useful for people who have the capacity to listen and truly *receive* the music; if a person does not have the capacity to focus on the music and experience it, receptive experiences are probably not the most appropriate to use.

Reminiscence can be very useful in the right situation, but the therapist must be prepared for unpleasant memories to arise. All of the memories are part of the client's life and can be dealt with productively. This does not mean that they should always be explored, though. While it is often helpful for a person to work through emotions elicited by the music, at times it is better to help the person contain a memory. This might occur if the person is too fragile or disturbed to deal with the feelings or if there is not enough support in the environment to help him or her to cope.

It is important to remember that not everyone finds the same music relaxing. For this reason, it is often a good idea to let the client select the music. However the music is chosen, it is important to observe the client's responses to determine whether the music is functioning as expected. If the music is not having the desired effect, the therapist should consider altering the music. The chapter "Selecting Music for Receptive Methods in Music Therapy" in Grocke and Wigram's (2007) book on receptive music therapy provides useful information on choosing music.

Materials

Music listening most often happens through playing a recorded version of the music, usually a CD. However, as you have learned in this chapter, the use of live music for receptive experiences is also a viable approach and is gaining increased recognition in recent years, particularly in neonatal intensive care units and other medical settings, as well as in hospice.

When using recorded music for receptive experiences, it is important that both the music recording and the equipment upon which it is played are of good quality. Although this requires budgeting extra money to purchase good equipment, it is money well spent. It is important that music—the tool of the music therapist—sounds good.

Music therapists should keep abreast of current technology. Advances in digital technology make this a rapidly changing area. Some of the vibroacoustic techniques involve specialized technology for which the therapist will need training. An additional consideration may be the high cost of technologically sophisticated equipment.

Anyone who is using music listening with clients will want to have a range of music for this purpose. For some ages, this can include music that has been collected over the years, but in the case of those who want to listen to current music, this needs to be constantly updated. Money will obviously need to be budgeted for this. Some music therapists feel that it is all right to use their personal music collections in working with clients. This does allow the therapist to continue using his or her music collection when moving to a different facility. While this can be beneficial, therapists should not hesitate to ask employers to pay for music. Music is an integral part of any music therapy program and should be supported.

It is also important to acquire music legally. Illegally downloaded or copied music should never be used in music therapy sessions (or by music therapists). Additionally, it is important to be aware of how the law affects the use of music in public spaces. More information about copyright can be found at www.copyright.gov.

Tips for Using

The choice of music is always important. Often, it makes the most sense to have clients choose the music that they want to hear. At other times, the therapist will want to choose the music, for example, if the client is unable to choose or if the therapist wants to elicit a particular mood or other targeted outcome. As discussed earlier, the therapist should observe the client's responses to be sure that they are as desired.

Inexperienced therapists may forget to check that a power source for a boom box will be available. This can be a cord and a working outlet, or working batteries. With technology changing all the time, it may be more likely that a therapist will be using a smartphone or iPad or other such tool for the provision of recorded music. The important thing is to make certain that your selections are cued up and your equipment is charged up! While many music therapists have probably made the mistake of not checking for a power cord or a fully charged battery prior to the session, it is unlikely that they make this mistake again, as it really hurts a session when the music isn't available!

Assignments—Receptive Experiences

Use these assignments to guide you in deepening your understanding of receptive experiences and how you might use them in your music therapy work:

- Describe a time when you observed a therapist using a receptive experience (a videotape or demonstration is okay). Based on the receptive experiences suggested by Bruscia (2014b) and described in the first two paragraphs of this chapter, are you able to identify the specific type of receptive experience that was implemented? What did you observe in the responses of the client(s) that could help the therapist to determine if the experience was beneficial?
- Think about incorporating the use of a receptive experience in one of your sessions. Considering the goals and objectives you already have identified for your client(s), is a receptive experience appropriate for addressing the goals? If so, how could you structure the intervention to include a receptive experience? Which type or types

of receptive experiences might be beneficial for your client(s)? How will you determine which type or types of receptive experiences to include, based on the anticipated benefits? How can you best prepare yourself to organize, present, develop, and process the experience?

- Find two examples of the use of receptive experiences with your current population in the literature; try to locate one example of use in individual therapy and another example of group work. Describe them and provide the sources.
- For the current client(s) you are observing and/or with whom you are working, ask your clinical supervisor to describe some possible applications of receptive experiences that have been or could be implemented. If receptive experiences have been used in previous sessions, how have the client(s) responded? If receptive experiences have not been used, is there a reason that they are contraindicated? Or, does your supervisor think that there could be benefits in providing such an experience? If so, are you able to participate in the development and/or presentation of a receptive experience?

12 Further Considerations in Planning

In this chapter, we will work with some of the ideas that were introduced in Chapter 4, The Process of Planning for Music Therapy. Here, however, we will go beyond our personal attitudes to consider the viewpoints of others. As you read this chapter, be sure to keep your earlier responses in mind; they will be very important as you integrate your own and others' ideas into a personal philosophy and style of working.

There are a number of things to consider as you begin to plan a session. All of these, of course, are aimed at developing a session that is most profitable for the clients. The result of all this planning will be a session with goals that meet the needs of the clients and procedures that are both effective and congruent with your values as a music therapist.

Characteristics of the Client

Music therapists should be aware of and comply with professional standards of practice. The AMTA *Standards of Clinical Practice* (American Music Therapy Association, 2013b) address the following areas: referral and acceptance, assessment, treatment planning, implementation, documentation, termination of services, continuing education, and supervision. Specific standards have also been adopted for the following areas: addictive disorders, consultant, intellectual and developmental disabilities, educational settings, older adults, medical settings, mental health, physical disabilities, private practice, and wellness.

Diagnosis

Some music therapists base much of their planning on the diagnosis of their clients, while others plan based only on the responses they observe in the session, without taking diagnoses into account.

Therapists who choose to take the diagnosis into consideration find that knowing the diagnosis and what it implies provides important information in planning for the needs of their clients. Certainly, knowledge of the diagnosis expands what the music therapist knows about the client, adding to the likelihood that the music therapy will be effective. It also provides some predictability about the client's behavior and a context for understanding what is occurring. For instance, if a client has a diagnosis of bipolar disorder, mixed type, the therapist knows that the person's mood may fluctuate between depressed and manic. Thus, when the client expresses varying moods during a session, the therapist is not surprised because he or she understands that the mood change was probably induced by the illness, not something that happened during the session. Similarly, the therapist realizes that a child with a diagnosis of attention deficit disorder is likely to have a short attention span and does not automatically assume that this occurs because of something being done wrong in the session.

This ability to anticipate possible responses and reactions is the very reason that some people feel that it is not helpful to know a client's diagnosis; they are concerned that therapists who know the diagnosis and thus anticipate certain responses will look for those types of reactions and not expect the client to achieve as much as might otherwise be possible.

While this is a reasonable concern, since there is so much to be gained from the knowledge of the client's diagnosis, a better solution seems to be to work to put aside the portion of that knowledge that would limit expectations. Certainly, it is important to expect as much as is both realistic and possible from our clients.

The *Diagnostic and Statistical Manual of Mental Disorders*, 5th edition (American Psychiatric Association, 2013), contains numerous diagnoses and their associated characteristics. It is important for music therapists to be familiar with this book, as it serves as a reference for psychiatric diagnostic information. Diagnoses are no longer made based on five axes, but instead are based on diagnostic categories, which are described in section 2 of the publication. A diagnosis is based on specific criteria outlined in the manual.

Three music therapy books are devoted exclusively to music therapy for clients with psychiatric disorders: *Music Therapy in the Treatment of Adults with Mental Disorders*, 2nd edition (Unkefer & Thaut, 2002); *Multimodal Psychiatric Music Therapy for Adults, Adolescents, and Children*, 3rd edition (Cassity & Cassity, 2006); and *Guidelines for Music Therapy Practice in Mental Health* (Eyre, 2013). These books provide a wealth of information for working with people with these difficulties.

Unkefer and Thaut (2002) and their collaborators provide suggestions of music therapy interventions based upon the diagnoses of adult clients with psychiatric difficulties. They have determined the major categories of adult emotional disorders that music therapists work with, including schizophrenic disorders; bipolar disorder, depressed episode; bipolar disorder, manic episode; and generalized anxiety disorder. For each category, they list the following: diagnostic symptoms, clinical features, characteristic behaviors, needs, music therapy interventions, programs, and techniques. For each diagnostic symptom, the additional categories are filled in, giving a number of symptom- and behavior-focused strategies for working with adults with emotional challenges.

Cassity and Cassity (2006) surveyed music therapy clinical training directors working in facilities treating people with psychiatric disorders. They asked the directors to select areas of nonmusic behavior that they assessed and treated most frequently during music therapy sessions. They then asked them to write two client problems that they assessed and treated most frequently for each of the selected areas. Finally, the directors were asked to list two music therapy interventions that they used most frequently to treat each of the client problems. The authors used Lazarus's (1976, 1989) Multimodal Therapy model to classify the problems and interventions. Following this model, the music therapy strategies address problems in the following areas: behavior, affect, sensation, imagery, cognitive, interpersonal, and drugs (this latter category encompasses any concerns about the client's state of health). The book presents an extensive collection of music therapy procedures for working on the problems specified by the clinical training directors, classified by the area addressed.

In special education settings, *classification* performs a function similar to that provided by diagnosis in psychiatric work. The classification systems in various states are based on federal regulations and are therefore similar, but with slight variations in terminology. Typical special education classifications include autism or autistic spectrum disorders, deaf-blindness, deafness, developmental delay, emotional disturbance, hearing impairment, intellectual disability, multiple disabilities, orthopedic impairment, other health impairment, specific learning disability, speech or language impairment, traumatic brain injury, and visual impairment, including blindness. These special education classifications apply to children ages 3 to 21.

It is important to understand the sequence of diagnosis and classification for children. When young children are seen for routine, well-child visits, one of the things that the pediatrician considers is whether the child is developing typically. This developmental monitoring is important in identifying *developmental delays* (included in the listing above). If delays are noted, developmental screening tests that can confirm this are performed; this is critical in supporting the family with early identification and early intervention. *Intellectual disability* (also listed above) refers to a variety of challenges that originate before the age of 18 and are characterized by significant difficulties in both intellectual functioning and adaptive behavior. Developmental disability (not included in the listing above) refers to severe disabilities that occur before the age of 22. Developmental disability encompasses intellectual disability but can also include physical disabilities. To learn more about these diagnoses and classifications, you may want to visit some of the following websites:

> American Association on Intellectual and Developmental Disabilities:
> https://aaidd.org/
> The Center for Parent Information and Resources:
> http://www.parentcenterhub.org/
> National Institutes of Health Fact Sheets:
> https://report.nih.gov/nihfactsheets/ViewFactSheet.aspx?csid=100

Developmental Level

It is useful for music therapists to know the developmental level at which their clients are functioning, which is often different from their chronological age. The importance of knowing the client's developmental level, particularly for children, is that this allows treatment plans to proceed in the logical order in which development naturally occurs. Even though children for whom music therapy is appropriate may not be developing in the expected order, interventions are often most effective if planned to meet developmental needs. This means that the new skills the therapist is helping the client to develop will be based on skills that the client has already achieved. This information may also be useful when working with adults who function at low developmental levels.

There are numerous approaches to understanding development. Piaget (Wadsworth, 1989) focuses on cognitive development; Freud (1938), on the role of psychosocial development in pathology; and Erikson (1950/1963), on psychosocial tasks that must be mastered at each stage of development, from infancy to old age. Behavioral theory (Skinner, 1976), attachment theory (Ainsworth & Bowlby, 1991; Schaeffer & Emerson, 1964), and social learning theory (Bandura, 1963) also contribute to our understanding of how children develop over time and can inform goal-setting, treatment planning, and implementation decisions within a session.

From a descriptive point of view, developmental charts are available that identify what a child can typically do at each age. These charts can be useful in learning to track childhood development and knowing what may be expected at different stages. It may be useful to keep one of these charts for reference. Numerous versions of developmental milestones charts are available on the Web. Dosman, Andrews, and Goulden (2012) provide a birth to age five developmental milestones chart that includes gross and fine motor skills, speech and language, and cognitive and social–emotional skills. Several things must be kept in mind when referring to these charts. One is that children develop at varying rates, so variations from the milestones listed are to be expected. Another is that, when children have developmental problems, as do many of the children seen in music therapy, their development is likely to be less even than that of children who are developing without specific delays. This means that they may work on or accomplish many developmental tasks in different orders than is considered typical or may seem to have mastered a task and then lose the skill, only to have to work on it again.

The best way to begin to really understand normal child development is to spend time around children who are developing without specific delays, as this helps the abstract behaviors shown on a chart to come alive.

Greenspan's Approach to Development

Greenspan's developmental framework (Greenspan, 1992; Greenspan & Wieder, 1998) can be very useful for music therapists. Greenspan and his colleagues find that children with developmental challenges frequently respond differently in three areas: (a) sensory reactivity, the way they take in information through the senses; (b) sensory processing, the way they make sense of the information they take in; and (c) muscle tone, motor planning, and sequencing, the way they use their bodies and later their thoughts to plan and execute responses to the information they have taken in (Greenspan & Wieder). They provide detailed information on assessing functioning in these areas in order to understand an individual child's reactions and to engage the child in interactions to aid in their development.

In their work with children, these clinicians have found that six types of emotional interactions correlate with six early phases of development and that "appropriate emotional experiences during each of these phases help develop critical cognitive, social, emotional, language, and motor skills, as well as a sense of self" (Greenspan & Wieder, 1998, p. 70). These milestones include:

- *Milestone I: Self-Regulation and Interest in the World.* In this phase, the infant learns to balance a growing awareness of sensations with the ability to remain calm. These researchers find that these skills are the most basic building blocks of emotional, social, and intellectual health. A child with difficulties in this area may cry and be upset because he or she is not able to regulate incoming sensations or be lethargic and appear lazy because not enough sensations are being perceived.
- *Milestone II: Intimacy.* In this phase, the child has learned to seek out the faces of the primary caregivers, to look them in the eye, and to smile, thus providing the building blocks for later relationships. A child who does not develop this ability (possibly due to problems in the previous stage) will not make adequate emotional connections with others, leading to a reduction in response from others, thus leading to increasing problems with intimacy.
- *Milestone III: Two-Way Communication.* This phase involves the *opening and closing of circles of communication.* For example, the child may smile at the mother and the mother smiles back in response, or the child reaches out to the father and the father reaches back to the child. From this, the child begins to learn that he or she can have an impact on the world. Children without this skill (possibly due to developmental problems in one of the above areas) will need extra assistance in learning to engage socially.
- *Milestone IV: Complex Communication.* The child in this phase has acquired gestures and, by linking them together, uses them as a vocabulary to express wishes. The child can therefore be clearer about what she or he is wanting and take initiatives in new ways. The child can also be more creative as he or she can express more complex thoughts. The child's sense of self builds as he or she engages in longer and longer conversations. These experiences with communication also establish the basis for speech.

- *Milestone V: Emotional Ideas.* In this stage, the child learns to express ideas first through play and then, through play, the increased use of words. Eventually, the child begins to realize that symbols stand for things, and with this comes awareness that words can communicate emotions. Eventually, the child learns to manipulate ideas and to use them in ways that meet his or her needs.
- *Milestone VI: Emotional Thinking.* The child in this stage begins to connect what were previously separate emotional thoughts, leading to the ability to express a wider range of emotions. Through this expression and expanded play, the child begins to understand more and more of what makes *me.* He or she becomes fully able to communicate ideas and feelings verbally.

The milestones are presented without any reference to age-specific achievement, since the children for whom they have been developed usually do not achieve them at the *normal* or expected age. Greenspan and his colleagues use these milestones as a framework to help parents and professionals understand what their children need and how to focus their work. This can serve as a framework for music therapists as well.

Carpente (2013) developed a method for working in music therapy based on Greenspan's theory (and in consultation with Greenspan) that he describes as a developmental relationship–based framework for assessing musical–play interactions. This way of working in music therapy focuses on how clients perceive, interpret, and create music with the therapist and is primarily an improvisational music–based relationship between the client and the therapist. This assessment may be used for developing treatment plans, to guide the therapist's musical decisions in working with the client, as a pre–post measure to evaluate client progress, and as a means of communicating information to the treatment team and/or caregivers. The tool is designed to evaluate clients (children and adults) with neurodevelopmental disorders at various developmental levels and chronological ages.

Developmental Stages in Adulthood

Erikson (1950/1963) described human growth and development in stages from birth to old age. As mentioned earlier, each stage includes a life task to be completed. Two stages are critical to adult functioning, adolescence and old age. In adolescence, the individual strives to develop an identity versus living with role confusion, and in late adulthood (up to age 80 years), the individual strives to find a sense of integrity versus living in despair. Feil (1980) developed a model for understanding adult development beyond Erikson's stages and added an additional stage, old-old age (80–100 years), with a life task of resolution versus vegetation. She posits that developmentally, "in old age, when controls loosen, disoriented very old persons are driven to express buried emotions in order to die in peace" (Feil, 2008, p. 797). She further defines stages of regression that appear in persons who do not resolve these emotions, including malorientation, time confusion, repetitive motion and vegetation, each with an accompanying life task (Feil, 2002). An understanding of these tasks and their accompanying body patterns, emotions, communication styles, and intellectual and memory rules can assist the music therapist when interacting with older adults experiencing these stages of development or regression and inform the choices made in music therapy treatment. Feil encourages the use of music with persons experiencing these regressive stages of development and recommends singing and movement to music as critical in addressing the emotional needs of the client.

Developmental Approaches to Music Therapy

Music in Developmental Therapy (Purvis & Samet, 1976) follows the outline of a curriculum that incorporates principles of development into special education (Wood, 1975; Wood, Quirk, & Swindle, 2007). Wood's *Developmental Therapy* sets goals for four areas of the curriculum: behavior, communication, socialization, and academic skills. Goals are established for each of five developmental stages under each of the four areas. Goals for each curriculum area at each stage of development are listed in Table 12.1. Purvis and Samet's (1976) book contains suggested learning experiences for a number of objectives under each goal and suggested music therapy procedures for achieving them. Although the book is out of print and may not be available to most music therapy students, the stages and areas can serve as a guide for formulating your own objectives and procedures.

Schwartz (2008) provides considerations for working with very young children in music, guidance into the world of how these children relate to music and how music therapists can use that relationship to enter into the world of the child. Working from theoretical models of musical development by Briggs (1991) and Briggs and Bruscia (1985), Schwartz outlines developmental levels of awareness, trust, independence, control, and responsibility and then demonstrates the correlation with the Briggs/Bruscia stages of musical development. Schwartz also provides examples of music therapy goals and objectives within each developmental level, along with specific music therapy strategies and interventions to address the goals and objectives.

In *Guidelines for Music Therapy Practice in Developmental Health,* edited by Hintz (2013b), experienced music therapists describe interventions for children with autism, speech and language delays, Rett syndrome, attention and learning disabilities, and behavioral, hearing, sight, and intellectual disabilities. Gooding and Standley (2011) have compiled information about musical development from the research literature and organized it by age. Their summary can be very helpful for music therapy students wishing to get a better grasp of musical development as it applies to their clients. Finally, Briggs (2015) provides a good overview of developmental issues as they relate to music and music therapy.

Needs of the Client

Level of Structure

One of the challenging but also fascinating qualities of music therapy is the breadth of its application. Music therapy can be used to elicit responses from a person in a coma or a child with multiple disabilities, just as Guided Imagery and Music or music psychotherapy can be used with high-functioning adults. Witnessing the power of music therapy to heal is one of the great rewards of being a music therapist. A qualitative research study by one of the authors on her pleasure in working with children with severe disabilities (Wheeler, 1999) is an excellent resource on this topic. The rewards are what keep many music therapists in the field but are not the subject of this chapter—it is the challenges that are being addressed here.

Music therapy clients vary widely in their level of functioning. Some need stimulation to elicit even the slightest response, while others have no clinical problems but are seeking higher levels of self-awareness or creativity. There are certain generalizations that may be made about clients at various levels, and these generalizations may be helpful in planning and treatment. One such generalization is that lower levels of function require greater structure, while higher levels require less structure. This applies to the psychotherapeutic framework used, to work at different developmental levels, and to work with varying diagnoses.

Table 12.1
Stages of Development in Developmental Therapy (Wood, 1975)
Used with permission from Mary M. Wood.

Stage	Behavior	Communication	Socialization	Academic Skills
I	to trust own body and skills	to use words to gain needs	to trust an adult sufficiently to respond to him	to respond to the environment with processes of classification, discrimination, basic receptive language concepts, and body coordination
II	to success-fully participate in routines and activities	to use words to affect others in constructive ways	to participate in activities with others	to participate in classroom routines with language concepts of similarities and differences, labels, use, color; numerical processes of ordering and classifying; and body coordination
III	to apply individual skills in group processes	to use words to express oneself in the group	to find satisfaction in group activities	to participate in the group with basic expressive language concepts; symbolic representation of experiences and concepts; functional, semi-concrete concepts of conservation; and body coordination

A continuum from directive to nondirective may be applied to the psychotherapeutic framework adopted by the music therapist. Some philosophies of therapy are more directive than others, leading music therapists embracing those philosophies to be more structured in their style of facilitating sessions. People practicing behavior modification, for instance, are likely to be more directive than those using some other approaches. A music therapist working to shape behaviors through the use of contingent music will be quite directive, for example, while a music therapist embracing a humanistic approach is likely to be less directive. A music therapist utilizing improvisation to explore feelings may be quite nondirective although directive on some occasions. It is not possible to make definitive statements about these styles, but it can be useful to be aware of these possibilities.

Levels of psychotherapy as they apply to music therapy have been conceptualized by several music therapists (Bruscia, 1998b; Maranto, 1993; Unkefer & Thaut, 2002; Wheeler, 1983, 1987a). A comparison of the classification by Wheeler with the one by Unkefer and Thaut is given in Table 12.2.

The concept of varying levels of structure also applies to developmental levels or levels of illness. Generally, developmental levels progress as children get older, such that older children are at higher developmental levels and thus require less structure. This also applies to clients with developmental problems. Older children at lower developmental levels are likely to need or be able to tolerate less structure as their developmental level advances. Developmental music therapy (Purvis & Samet, 1976) takes into account this advancing need for less structure, where suggested activities at higher stages include less structure than those at lower levels.

Hadsell (1993) proposes three levels of external structure for music therapy clients and suggests procedures for providing structure in the areas of time, space and equipment, choices, materials, instructions, and activities. Her suggestions are summarized in Table 12.3.

The level of structure needed has also been linked to diagnoses. The works of Wheeler (1983, 1987a) and Unkefer and Thaut (2002) describe the correlation between the level of structure required in a session and the level of personality organization of the client. Thus, those with diagnoses associated with more primitive personality organization benefit from more structured music therapy sessions. Unkefer and Thaut have also suggested clients and problems for which each level of psychotherapeutic intervention is appropriate. Clients suggested as appropriate for each level are outlined in Table 12.4.

Table 12.2
Levels of Music Therapy Practice (Unkefer & Thaut, 2002; Wheeler, 1983, 1987a; Wolberg, 1977)

	Wheeler (based on Wolberg)	**Unkefer & Thaut**
First Level	**MT as Activity Therapy** Goals achieved through use of therapeutic activities (including verbalization when appropriate); understanding why a behavior occurs is not considered important.	**Supportive, Activities-Oriented MT** Goals achieved through active involvement in therapeutic activities; any verbal processing focuses on here-and-now and overt behavior during session; activities aimed at strengthening defenses, supporting healthy feelings and thoughts, developing appropriate mechanisms of behavior control, reassuring reality stimulation; activities tightly structured to promote success, support, reduction of anxiety.
Second Level	**Insight MT with Re-educative Goals** Music may be used to elicit certain emotional and/or cognitive reactions necessary for the therapy. The major focus is on feelings, the exposition and discussion of which lead to insight, resulting in improved functioning.	**Re-educative, Insight, and Process-Oriented MT** Active involvement in therapy is complemented by verbalization; activities are designed for feelings and thoughts that are then subjected to verbal processing within therapy session; therapeutic emphasis is on exposition of personal thoughts, feelings, and interpersonal reaction; focus of attention is on here-and-now of the interactional process between MT and clients; aimed at helping client to reorganize values and behavioral patterns, to acquire new tension- and anxiety-relieving interpersonal attitudes.
Third Level	**Insight MT with Reconstructive Goals** MT elicits unconscious material, which is then worked with in an effort to promote reorganization of the personality.	**Reconstructive, Analytically, and Catharsis-Oriented MT** Therapeutic activities are utilized to uncover, relive, and resolve unconscious conflicts; unconscious material is elicited, then used to reorganize the personality by living through, with insight, deepest fears and conflicts.

Table 12.3
Levels of External Structure in Music Therapy (Hadsell, 1993)
Used with permission from the American Music Therapy Association.

Level	Time	Space/ Equipment	Choices	Materials	Instructions	Activities
One (maximum)	Specific time allotted for each activity; consistent sequence; minimal time between activities	MT controls; each item or activity occupies a specific space, unchanged from session to session; consistent use of equipment	Initially no options given, later two choices; therapist determines choices based on assessment of client preferences	MT creates materials to support objectives; items constructed for sturdiness; materials placed so therapist has control	MT gives 1- or 2-step instructions; may be written or illustrated with pictures; MT may demonstrate desired responses	Conducted step by step to elicit highly structured, simple responses; desired behaviors task-analyzed into careful sequences
Two (moderate)	Scheduled activities during sessions generally have allotted times and sequences, but with some variation; client input considered in planning	MT controls use of space and equipment but can vary from session to session; space rearranged by MT as needs change; client requests included in planning	MT gives several options to clients; clients may have limited direct input into alternatives offered	May be numerous and varied to address similar objectives; clients may help to create by stating preferences; may help in caring for objects, leading to more available materials	MT may give simple to moderately complex instructions with several sequential response levels; written instructions may be used in step-by-step format; MT demonstrates as needed	Activities are designed to elicit moderately complex responses; fewer steps needed than at previous level; tasks may not be specifically analyzed, since clients may master several small steps at once
Three (minimum)	Session time is loosely scheduled; flexibility built into planning; activities can take varying time as needed	Space used flexibly with equipment and materials placed for mobility; items easily accessible to clients; clients and MT can rearrange room as necessary	MT offers options; MT and clients work together to devise alternatives consistent with therapeutic objectives; questions of preference may be open-ended	Clients may collaborate with MT in creation of appropriate materials; clients have access to materials and may be responsible for bringing them to sessions	MT may give complex verbal or written instructions; clients may request clarification through explanation or demonstrations; language level varies	Activities may be planned by both MT and clients; both may decide on steps needed to complete objectives; steps may be arranged for greater effectiveness

Table 12.4
Levels of Music Therapy Practice and Clients Appropriate for Each Level (Unkefer & Thaut, 2002; Wheeler, 1983, 1997a)

	Wheeler	Unkefer & Thaut
First Level	**Music Therapy as Activity Therapy** Appropriate for most seriously ill clients or those with the most serious personality disorganization; could include those hospitalized for psychiatric disorders or people with chronic schizophrenia in long-term community treatment (research confirmed use with people with schizophrenia)	**Supportive, Activities-Oriented Music Therapy** Appropriate for clients who have basically sound ego structures who have broken down temporarily under stress; for acute or chronic clients who are fragmented, regressed, or delusional, who suffer from severe schizophrenic, affective, or organic symptoms, or who are too phobic and anxious to participate in more demanding levels of therapy; these clients need support, integration, and *sealing over* rather than verbal investigation of their problems
Second Level	**Insight Music Therapy with Re-educative Goals** Appropriate for clients whose problems do not cause severe personality disorganization, such as substance abusers, people with affective disorders, neuroses/anxiety disorders, situational disorders, or personality disorders; or for those with schizophrenia if used over a longer period of time (research confirmed use with those who abuse substance; people with affective disorders, neuroses, personality disorders)	**Re-educative, Insight, and Process-Oriented Music Therapy** Appropriate for clients who are willing and able to self-disclose; helps clients to reorganize values and behavioral patterns, to acquire new tension- and anxiety-relieving interpersonal attitudes, and, through projection of personal thoughts and feelings in the therapy process, to learn to assume responsibility for them
Third Level	**Insight Music Therapy with Reconstructive Goals** Appropriate for clients whose problems do not cause severe personality disorganization, as above, and for healthy people desiring additional growth (research confirmed use with those who abuse substances, people with affective disorders, neuroses, personality disorders, situational disorders)	**Reconstructive, Analytically, and Catharsis-Oriented Music Therapy** Appropriate for clients who are able and motivated to commit themselves to long-term therapy that challenges existent personality structures

The Music Therapist's Perspective

It is essential for you as a music therapist to know *why* you are doing what you are doing. We will discuss various aspects of this, beginning with the personal theory of helping and then expanding our understanding to include what has been said by others and incorporating it into the development of our own theory. We will then apply all of these to clarifying the rationale for our music therapy plans and treatment.

Personal Theory of Helping

The ideas that you considered in Chapter 4 have been formulated into your personal theory of helping. This theory will help you in many ways, serving as a guide in making many decisions about therapy. It will be revised over time as you mature and your views change.

Your theory of helping may also embrace the philosophy embodied in one or more psychotherapeutic frameworks or be part of a framework based on an indigenous model of music therapy. To see what others say about these areas, we will now look at how others—music therapists, psychologists, psychotherapists—have formulated and used theories. These will include those who see music therapy as part of a psychotherapeutic framework and those who have developed a theory of music therapy separate from psychotherapeutic theories.

Psychotherapeutic Framework

A therapist who embraces behavior modification as a theory will plan a session differently than one who employs a psychodynamic framework. Just as psychotherapists use varying frameworks for their work, so do music therapists. It is useful to be familiar with various psychotherapeutic frameworks and to draw from one or more in one's music therapy work.

Ruud (1980) examines the psychological orientations of psychoanalytic, behavioral, and humanistic/existential approaches and the music therapy theories derived from each, drawing parallels between music therapists and others who employ the theoretical frameworks. Others (Bruscia, 1987; Darrow, 2008; Wheeler, 1981) have related music therapy to a variety of psychotherapeutic frameworks. Some authors have done extensive analyses of aspects of music therapy within a single psychotherapeutic framework. Examples of this are a book by Madsen (1980) on the use of music therapy and behavior modification with people with intellectual and developmental disabilities and one edited by Bruscia (1998b) on aspects of music therapy within a psychodynamic framework.

Music Therapy Theoretical Framework

Some music therapists (Aigen, 1991; Amir, 1996; Kenny, 1985, 1989) argue that music therapists should not rely on a framework based on psychotherapy but instead need to have a framework based on an indigenous model of music therapy itself. These authors have written on a variety of aspects addressing this area.

Although as a music therapist just developing your clinical skills it is unlikely that you will be ready to focus on the development of theory, now is a good time to start thinking about some questions that may later lead to theory development. A theory is defined by Bruscia (2014b) as

> a set of interrelated ideas, formulated or discerned by a theorist to: (a) identify, organize, and interpret knowledge on a particular domain; (b)

explain or understand related facts, empirical data, and phenomena within the domain; and (c) offer a conceptual framework for decision-making in future theory, research, and practice. (p. 199)

Having a theory is like having a map to guide us to a chosen destination. A theory in music therapy serves as a guide as we determine how to conduct our music therapy sessions.

Although we don't usually think about it, we each use theories to guide us through many aspects of our lives. One way to discover how we use a theory is when something doesn't work—perhaps a light won't turn on. If our first action is to pull the cord or to flip the switch again, the guiding thought (a theory) is that something didn't catch the first time. If this doesn't work, we may test another theory—that the light bulb is broken. (This is an example of using a theory to form a hypothesis that we then test.) If the light comes on once a new bulb is installed, our hypothesis has been confirmed and our theory appears to be correct. If it does not come on, our theory needs revision. Perhaps the next theory is that the light fixture is broken.

To begin to develop theory in music therapy, we follow a similar process. Carolyn Kenny suggested the following steps:

We might initially reflect on our "underlying assumptions." This is a good way to begin the theoretical thinking. The next step, I believe, is to have them design "principles." These are "if, then" statements. Try to do this with complete honesty, even if your principles seem "unfounded" or "unsupported." It is good to get these out in the open and to relate the principles to the underlying assumptions. The next step from the principles is "concept formation," and the next is to develop a "set of concepts." Finally comes the map, or how the concepts relate to each other. At this point, you have your theory. Remember that theories are guides or maps. You don't have to use your theory to "prove" that you are right, though you can take that next step if you decide to do research in a positivistic paradigm. (personal communication, July 20, 2001)

You may also wish to read what Kenny wrote about theory development in "The Field of Play" (2006, pp. 86–92). A comprehensive overview of the development of theory in music therapy by Bruscia (2005) provides additional information on this topic.

Rationale for Treatment

According to Merriam-Webster (www.merriam-webster.com/dictionary/rationale, 2016), a *rationale* is "an explanation of controlling principles of opinion, belief, practice, or phenomena; an underlying reason; basis."

Your rationale for what you are doing is most useful if it reflects your overall way of viewing therapy and change and takes into account various aspects of the therapy. The rationale will generally be developed prior to and as a part of learning to work with clients. Knowing *why* you are doing what you are doing is a step that is often neglected, particularly in the early stages of learning to do music therapy. Too often, students and beginning therapists know what they want to do—which strategy to use—but don't know why. The rationale is influenced by the therapist's personal theory of helping as well as by psychotherapy- or music therapy-based theoretical frameworks adopted by the therapist.

As a student music therapist, you should always have a rationale for what you are doing with clients. This rationale will take into account much of what we have looked at so far—the needs of the client, your personal feelings, your philosophy of helping and the psychotherapeutic and other theoretical frameworks that you adopt, your understanding of the role of music in the treatment. The rationale may easily change as the situation changes. The rationale helps you to make decisions minute by minute during the session and is something that you might tell someone—perhaps a parent or another professional—should they ask why you are doing something.

Questions that arise in developing a rationale for a particular intervention or approach include the following: What does the client need? What does the group need? What has been done before? How much time is available in the session? How many more sessions are likely to take place? The rationale is most likely to develop from the answers to questions like this and will probably encompass several of the answers. While it is possible to conduct music therapy without a rationale, sessions that are based on a solid rationale are most likely to be productive.

Ethical Considerations

The music therapist must follow ethical standards in all areas of functioning, including planning and carrying out sessions. This includes both personal and professional ethics. Being aware of one's personal values and ethical standards is part of developing as an ethical professional. Professional ethics are based upon personal ethics as well as more generally accepted professional ethical standards.

Ethical standards have been developed over a period of years and cover many areas. Most professions have adopted statements of ethical standards. The AMTA *Code of Ethics* (American Music Therapy Association, 2014a) covers the following general areas: professional competence and responsibilities; general standards; relationships with clients/students/research subjects; relationships with colleagues; relationship with employers; responsibility to community/public; responsibility to the profession/association; research; fees and commercial activities; announcing services; education (teaching, supervision, administration); and implementation. Students and professional music therapists should follow it in their professional activities and consult it when they have questions about ethical behavior in specific situations. Since the guidelines are general, there will undoubtedly be times when they do not address a specific situation. At these times, it is a good idea to discuss the situation with a teacher, supervisor, or colleague. *Ethical Thinking in Music Therapy* by Dileo (2000) is a valuable resource when considering ethical issues. This book will challenge you to examine your understanding of ethics and provides a step-by-step process for addressing ethical concerns in your daily work.

Other music therapy associations also have codes of ethics, and the Certification Board for Music Therapists (CBMT) has developed a *Code of Professional Practice* (2011). Although this document applies only to board-certified music therapists, as a student on the path to becoming a credentialed professional, you can benefit from its guidance on professional standards in your chosen field of practice.

In addition, the AMTA and CBMT collaborated on the creation of the *Scope of Music Therapy Practice* (American Music Therapy Association, 2015b; Certification Board for Music Therapists, 2015b). As indicated on the CBMT website:

> The Scope of Music Therapy Practice (2015) broadly defines the range of responsibilities of a fully qualified music therapy professional with requisite education, clinical training, and board certification. Created and approved by AMTA and CBMT, this document considers the contributions, interrelationships, and interdependencies of the CBMT Scope of Practice

(2010) & Code of Professional Practice, as well as the AMTA Standards of Clinical Practice, Professional Competencies, & Code of Ethics. (n.p.)

Assignments—Further Considerations in Planning

The following exercises should help to deepen your understanding of these considerations in planning:

- Based on the charts, IEPs, and *DSM-5* or other appropriate sources, write about the characteristics of the people in your music therapy session. Provide the rationale for your session plans and outcomes, making connections between the characteristics of the clients and what you are doing in the session.
- Speak with a music therapist or another professional where you are doing your clinical work about one of the clients with whom you are involved. Find out the diagnosis and some of the characteristics that led to that diagnosis. Write the behaviors that you observe that you think might be associated with this diagnosis.
- Look at the general AMTA *Standards of Practice.* Choose any three of the standards and reflect on why they exist and how they might apply to your population.
- Examine the appropriate level of structure for your group and/or individual client, using Tables 12.2 and 12.3. For each, determine where your work falls and write about this, describing your reasons for placing it where you do.
- List the behaviors and/or responses that a client in your current practicum placement is exhibiting and relate them to one of the developmental frameworks presented (a list of developmental tasks, Greenspan, or Developmental Therapy).
- Relate the music therapy that you are doing to your theory of helping, adding information from what others have written about helping (psychotherapeutic or music therapy theories).
- Reread Kenny's steps in theory development and use them as a guide to begin to formulate your own theory of music therapy. Discuss this with a peer or your site supervisor or instructor.

13 Facilitating Client Responses

Music therapists help people to make many types of changes. Music therapy treatment may lead to changes in behavior, changes in self-awareness, changes in skills (such as communication, social, leisure, motor), changes in self-management (such as stress, pain, emotions), or changes in understanding the world in which we live. Sometimes we help people to gain insights that may later lead to changes of behavior. At other times, we help clients to modify their behavior more directly.

Music therapists use various means of eliciting client responses, with some differences between the techniques used with lower- and higher-functioning clients. With lower-functioning clients, responses may be elicited through music, through physical prompts, and through verbal prompts. Many of the same techniques are used with higher-functioning clients, but talking becomes more important since these people tend to be more verbal.

Verbal Facilitation

We each have ways in which we typically interact with others, so it is natural that our verbal facilitation as therapists will in part be built upon this interaction style. However, our natural or habitual responses become problematic if they dominate our interactions, if we are unaware of them and their impact, or if we cannot move out of a particular style of interacting when the situation calls for it. Part of our training as music therapists, therefore, is to learn different ways of interacting and their likely impact—positive or negative—and then to practice moving smoothly and skillfully from one style of interaction to another. In time, we will be able to manage our interactions effectively to facilitate our clients' growth. Of course, since people do not always respond as we expect them to, we should always be ready for surprises.

Therapist Responses That Are Helpful

Verbal techniques and responses may be divided into categories in different ways, most of which deal with their typical uses and effects. The categories described below, which may be used by verbal therapists as well as music therapists, are followed by music therapy examples.

Encouraging Communication and Gathering Information

The therapist may use several types of questions to encourage the client to communicate. When asking questions, it is most helpful for the therapist to use questions that cannot be answered with a simple "yes" or "no." During this process, active listening and conveying understanding form the foundation of a therapist's role with clients. The therapist responds not only to the verbal content, but also to the client's total message, including nonverbal behaviors such as body language, voice inflection and volume, breathing patterns, and so on. Listening and understanding also involve letting clients know that you are aware of them and what they are saying by making eye contact and indicating your understanding through your own facial and body gestures. Verbal skills for listening and understanding include *paraphrasing,* in which the client's basic message is stated in similar, but usually fewer, words. The therapist may also use *clarifying,* attempting to restate what the client is saying or asking the client to clarify, repeat, or illustrate what was being said. In general, questions should be used sparingly, as they tend to put the client on the spot and keep the therapist in a central position. The therapist may use a leading question to help the client begin, for example, "What would you like to talk about today?" or "Tell me more about what happened in that situation."

A music therapist may use the same types of questions to encourage communication. When beginning a session, the therapist may ask, "Is there anything left from last week's session that we need to complete?" or "What music would you like to start with today?" Either of these questions may be answered verbally or, perhaps after a brief verbal response, musically. A similar question that would lead straight into music would be, "Does anyone have an image that they would like to share through the instruments as we begin our group?"

Reflecting and Sharing

When the therapist reflects, he or she is attempting to communicate his or her perception of the client's world as the client sees it. Feelings or content may be reflected. When the therapist reflects feelings, he or she uses different words than the client was using to express those feelings. Reflecting content is similar to paraphrasing. By reflecting the content of what has been said or of a client's feelings or experience, the therapist is helping the client to find the words to express him- or herself.

When the therapist recognizes that she or he is having a feeling, it is often useful to express it to the client. It is helpful if the therapist can separate his or her own personal issues from the normal human response to the client's presentation or issues; it is the latter feelings that are often helpful to express. This area deals with the therapist's countertransferences, or personal associations, that are affecting his or her responses to the client. The therapist may also describe and share feelings to serve as a model for the client.

Both the reflecting of the client's feelings and the sharing of the therapist's feelings may occur in music therapy. For example, a therapist who is working with a group of children and notes that several of them are feeling angry but may not know how to express the feeling might say, "I wonder if some of us are feeling angry about what just occurred. We can talk about our anger or play it on the instruments, as long as we don't hurt anyone or the instruments. This might help us feel better." Or, the therapist may share his or her own feelings about something that is occurring, perhaps saying, "When I see people crying because their feelings have been hurt, I feel like crying, too, or I find some music to play or listen to that helps me express my sadness." This is likely to help the children to see that their feelings are acceptable and to provide a model for how to deal with them.

There are other times when it is helpful to share information with a client, for example, factual information that therapists know (not necessarily because they are therapists) that clients may need to know. There are also times when advice may be shared, although we recommend that it be given sparingly. If advice is given, it should be based on solid expertise and given in the form of tentative suggestions.

Information or advice specific to music therapy involves sharing musical information. A music therapist may share information about how to use music as a coping skill with a medical patient. This may follow a music-assisted relaxation experience in a session. The music therapist shares information for the purpose of assisting the patient in making a plan for using music at home to manage pain or anxiety. Another example might be sharing information about the types of CD players or keyboards with a client who is preparing to buy one of these. For these latter situations, the music therapist is likely to have unique knowledge and experience that is certainly helpful and appropriate to share, although doing so probably has minimal, if any, therapeutic value.

Interpreting

Interpreting involves an attempt to make sense of something about the client, the client's life, or the therapeutic process. This may be done by the therapist, the client, or the therapist and the client together. When defined in this way, interpreting is another word for finding meaning or making sense of something that the client says or does. It is important to realize that this is a central undertaking in many types of music therapy. Goals of interpreting are to help clients learn how to interpret their own feelings, expressions, and behavior while also bringing them insights into themselves and their lives. Interpretations are most helpful when they reflect both the client's and the therapist's points of view and when the therapist presents the interpretation in a sensitive manner when the client is ready to receive and understand it. When interpretations are wrong, or when the therapist does not present them in a sensitive, timely way, they create distance between the client and therapist and may evoke negative feelings.

Interpretation in therapy is an art that requires considerable knowledge and skill on the part of the therapist. Sometimes the therapist's interpretations can also be based on a particular treatment orientation (such as psychodynamic) or music therapy model (such as Analytical Music Therapy [AMT] or the Bonny Method of Guided Imagery and Music [BMGIM]), all of which require additional, specialized training. Many examples of interpreting occur in music therapy within a psychodynamic framework (see Ahonen-Eerikäinen, 2007; Bruscia, 1998b; Hadley, 2003), using AMT (Eschen, 2002; Priestley, 1994) or BMGIM (Bruscia & Grocke, 2002), and in other approaches that follow particular theories.

Confronting and Providing Feedback

There may be times when it is helpful for the therapist to give the client feedback. Feedback can be useful when the client has asked for it or accepted the therapist's offer of feedback. It should be clear that the feedback is given on the client's behavior rather than as a judgment on the client him- or herself. It is also important to give feedback in small doses and to discuss the client's reaction after it has been given.

At other times, the therapist will want to confront the client or challenge his or her perceptions or behavior. These techniques are more forceful than simple feedback and are often most effective when the client trusts the therapist. They should be used only when necessary. In general, it is better for the client's ideas to emerge from the client's own process than from the therapist.

Music therapists may find situations in which giving feedback or confronting is useful. For instance, a music therapist may be working with a client who repeatedly states that he wants to learn a precomposed piece for resonator bars to present as a musical gift to his family during the upcoming holiday season. However, he repeatedly refuses to work on his selected piece in therapy, and, when pushed to do so, he throws the mallets and walks out of the session. Perhaps the therapist and others on the treatment team have worked with the client to increase his awareness of his avoidance behavior and to help him in a variety of ways to change it. The music therapist may decide that the most effective technique is to confront the client about his behavior the next time that it occurs in music therapy. For example, the client refuses the opportunity to play resonator bars in a session, even in a free improvisation. To confront the client, the music therapist might intervene with, "This is an example of how you avoid responsibility and resist following through on your goals. If you really want to share your music with your family, you need to practice playing the resonator bars and start working on learning your chosen piece." This direct confrontation could lead to a discussion with the client, perhaps including efforts to engage him in creating some sort of color-coded music chart to help him feel more confident in beginning this process. A less direct response to a similar situation might be to give feedback. The music therapist might say, "We need to talk about why you keep refusing to work on your piece. If we don't figure out a way to work on this soon you won't be ready by the holidays. How can we make this easier for you?" This feedback also includes a suggestion of a collaborative strategy or solution, perhaps relieving some of the perceived pressure or issues with self-confidence and self-esteem with which the client might be struggling.

Therapist Responses That Are Not Helpful

Bolton (1979) describes barriers to communication in three categories: judgment, sending solutions, and avoidance of the other's concerns. We are presenting these here so that music therapy students will be aware of these pitfalls and avoid them. When things do not go well in a session, it can be useful to reflect on whether you inadvertently put up of one of these barriers.

It is important to note that some of these specific responses (e.g., diagnosing if you are not licensed to do so) go beyond being *not helpful* and may be considered illegal. Some are actually identified as forms of abuse (e.g., criticizing, name-calling, and threatening are generally considered to be forms of psychological abuse).

Judgment

Some therapist techniques may lead to a client feeling judged. There are times when we, as humans, *do* feel judgmental of people, whether we encounter these people in our daily activities or in our work as music therapists. When this happens, we should remember that our role as therapists is not to judge, and we should do our best not to judge our clients. In addition, we need to look into ourselves to see where these reactions, a form of countertransference, are coming from. Judgments include the following:

- *Criticizing:* Making a negative evaluation of the other person, his or her actions, or attitudes.
- *Name-calling:* Putting down or stereotyping the other person.
- *Diagnosing:* Analyzing why a person is behaving as he or she is; playing amateur psychiatrist.
- *Praising evaluatively:* Making a positive judgment of the other person, his or her actions, or attitudes.

Sending Solutions

In most therapeutic situations, our role is to help the client find solutions, not to impose our own solutions. Examples of sending solutions are listed below:

- *Ordering:* Commanding the other person to do what you want to have done.
- *Threatening:* Trying to control the other's actions by warning of negative consequences that you will instigate.

- *Moralizing:* Telling another person what he or she *should* do; preaching at the other.
- *Excessive or inappropriate questioning:* Closed-ended questions are often barriers in a relationship; these are those that can usually be answered in a few words—often with a simple yes or no.
- *Advising:* Giving the other person a solution to his or her problems.

Avoidance of the Other's Concerns

As therapists, we must remember that the concerns that the client presents are the focus of the therapy, regardless of whether we feel that they are important or can be dealt with. The important thing is that they are important to the client. The following are ways in which a therapist may avoid the concerns of the client:

- *Diverting:* Pushing the other's problems aside through distraction.
- *Logical argument:* Attempting to convince the other with an appeal to facts or logic, usually without consideration of the emotional factors involved.
- *Reassuring:* Trying to stop the other person from feeling the negative emotions that he or she is experiencing.

In your studies, you are learning about verbal facilitation through many other resources, so there is no need to delve into further detail in this book. Many books and other resources provide information on aspects of verbal facilitation. Among those that we recommend are *The Helping Relationship: Process and Skills,* 8th edition, by Brammer and MacDonald (2003); *Becoming a Helper,* 7th edition, by Corey and Corey (2015); *Current Psychotherapies,* 8th edition, by Corsini and Wedding (2007); and *Intentional Interviewing and Counseling: Facilitating Client Development in a Multicultural Society,* 8th edition, by Ivey, Ivey, and Zalaquett (2014).

The use of verbal techniques in music therapy should be driven by an awareness of the needs of the client. Is the individual able to participate in verbal interaction, or can they only engage receptively? Would the use of discussion be a beneficial complement to musical interaction, or would it perhaps be a distraction? Make certain that you are using verbal techniques because they are called for in the clinical moment, to help move the therapeutic process forward, and not because you are uncertain of how to proceed musically.

As music therapists, even when working with clients who are highly verbal, we must not lose sight of the power of our primary tool: music. It is our unique contribution to the client's treatment, and too often we underestimate the impact and value it holds. Sometimes, we may even find ourselves forgetting the significance of music in our work and in the lives of our clients. Bruscia related a story at a conference presentation in 1984. He shared the case of a young man who had suffered a traumatic brain injury, resulting in the loss of speech. The treatment team determined that a primary goal for this client was to regain expressive language, and all team members, including the music therapist, were to concentrate on this area of rehabilitation. After months of therapy (including music therapy, speech therapy, and other services), the client was clearly becoming frustrated with the overriding focus on having him produce language. When the focus of music therapy became that of nonverbal communication through musical improvisation, the changes in the client were significant. The message for us as music therapists is clear: Do not ever underestimate the power of music in the lives of the people we serve.

Musical Facilitation

Since much of what music therapists do deals with nonverbal behavior, including musical responses, music therapists must be proficient at responding nonverbally. There are a range of strategies for use in nonverbal facilitation. They can broadly be categorized into two distinct areas: body language (including facial expressions, eye contact, movement, etc.) and physical proximity. Consideration should also be given to the use of silence versus vocal response (e.g., "uh-huh"). Even the way you dress for your sessions and distracting habits you may have (Do you begin every other sentence with "yeah" or "um"? Do you push your hair behind your ears when you are nervous?) can be considered forms of nonverbal communication that can enhance or diminish your efforts with nonverbal facilitation. We are focusing this section on a particular type of nonverbal facilitation in which music therapists are uniquely qualified, musical facilitation.

Bruscia (1987) identifies 64 clinical techniques utilized in improvisational music therapy, most of which are nonverbal. He classified the specific techniques into nine distinct groupings: techniques of empathy, structuring techniques, techniques of intimacy, elicitation techniques, redirection techniques, procedural techniques, emotional exploration techniques, referential techniques, and discussion techniques. Many of his discussion techniques align with some of the verbal facilitation techniques mentioned earlier in this chapter. Here are some examples:

- *Encouraging communication and gathering information* is similar to Bruscia's discussion techniques of *probing* (asking questions to elicit information) and *clarifying* (getting the client to verify information that has been offered);
- *Reflecting and sharing* is comparable to Bruscia's discussion technique of *disclosing* (wherein the therapist reveals something personal to the client during a session);
- *Interpreting* is similar to Bruscia's discussion technique of the same name, *interpreting* (providing possible explanations for certain experiences of the client);
- *Confronting and providing feedback* is similar to Bruscia's discussion techniques of *confronting* (pointing out possible contradictions in the client's responses) and *feedback* (stating how the client might appear).

While many of the techniques (such as *imitating, repeating, completing, calming,* and *pausing*) in the other groupings may appear to be verbal techniques based on what they are called and could indeed be implemented verbally, Bruscia presents them as musical techniques, providing brief as well as more detailed descriptions of how to implement the techniques and identifying specific clinical outcomes toward which each may be most applicable. Remember that these techniques are specifically identified and described within an improvisational context and that they are more often used in combinations rather than in isolation. A brief summary of the remaining groupings, as stated above, is offered.

When implementing *techniques of empathy*, the therapist may imitate or synchronize with what the client is doing or match the client's energy level. The therapist may also try to express through his or her music the same mood or emotion that the client is expressing or may exaggerate something distinctive about the client's response.

Structuring techniques are utilized when the therapist strives to establish rhythmic stability by providing a stable beat or a tonal center or harmonic ground for the client's improvising, as well as helping to define phrasing.

Techniques of intimacy include having the therapist share instruments with the client or provide a musical gift such as a performance. The therapist may develop a short piece that serves as a theme for the relationship and may at times create lyrical improvisations as if talking to him- or herself about the client.

Elicitation techniques provide opportunities for the therapist to model certain skills for the client to imitate or to present a repeating rhythm or melody, encouraging a similar response from the client. After a structure (rhythmic, melodic, lyrical, etc.) is established, the therapist may leave spaces within the structure in which the client can respond or, in contrast, may wait for a break in the client's improvisation and fill in the gap. The therapist may establish a musical question-and-answer or turn-taking structure within the improvisation or extend the client's response by adding something to the end of it.

When implementing *redirection techniques*, the therapist may introduce changes in the music (rhythmically, melodically, lyrically, tonally, metered) or play music that is different yet compatible with the client's music. Increasing or decreasing the dynamics, tempo, or rhythmic or melodic tension of the improvisation may regain the client's focus, as can interrupting or presenting instability.

Procedural techniques are indicated when the therapist decides to institute more instructional approaches, having the client shift from one modality to another or having him or her pause at specific points in the improvisation. The therapist may provide a general structure and have the client experiment with improvising within the structure, or the therapist may assume the role of conductor and even have the client rehearse a particular improvisation and then perform and or record it.

Referential techniques may be effective in establishing context and carryover. The therapist may pair different musical motifs with specific client responses each time they occur in a session. The therapist may suggest that the client use something musical to represent something else or have the client recall a particular event and reproduce it in an improvisation. Free association exercises, fantasizing, and storytelling can also be introduced.

Finally, *emotional exploration techniques* are indicated when the therapist works to provide opportunities for the client to explore and expand his or her range of emotional experience. The therapist may improvise in such a way as to contain the client's feelings as they improvise together or to express feelings that the client is struggling to acknowledge. The therapist may have the client explore emotions by improvising opposite feelings and then find ways within an improvisation to move from one type of feeling to its opposite. The therapist may suggest that the client put components of an improvisation in a particular sequence or swap various roles with the therapist while improvising.

Expressive Elements of Music

We have discussed verbal facilitation techniques and musical clinical facilitation techniques. But how do you decide what music to use, what form of presentation to implement (such as live or recorded, precomposed or improvised, vocal or instrumental, and so on), and how to actually have music function as an essential facilitator in music therapy sessions? Concentrate for a moment on why you are reading this book: You are in the process of becoming a music therapist. A *music* therapist. You are already a musician, becoming a therapist. What do you know about music? What are the essential elements of music that make it an expressive medium? Rhythm, melody, harmony, and form are considered to be the building blocks of music; they are sometimes referred to as the constituent elements of music. Other primary components of music include texture, tempo, and dynamics. Wigram (2004), in discussing musical elements, identifies "core elements of music: pitch/frequency, tempo/pulse, rhythm, intensity/volume, duration, melody, and harmony" (p. 35). Aigen (2014a), in describing aspects of music-centered music therapy and the origins of the Nordoff-Robbins approach, touches on many of the expressive elements already mentioned, as well as others, including tonality, timbre, touch, style, and the incorporation of movement and lyrics. Additional elements include things such as phrasing, repetition, ornamentation, meter, and so on.

As a music therapist, it is critical that you nurture and develop your musicianship and your theoretical understanding of music and all of its elements; only through this sort of concentrated effort will you be able to provide a rich musical experience for your clients, having a well-stocked toolkit of musical elements and resources from which to draw upon. Outstanding musicianship blended with clinical skills and therapeutic insight will enable you to be the best music therapist you can be for every person with whom you work.

Assignments—Facilitating Client Responses

These assignments will assist you in deepening your understanding of verbal and musical facilitation techniques:

- Think about sessions in which you have observed and assisted. Recall if any of the verbal facilitation responses listed in this chapter (encouraging communication and gathering information; reflecting and sharing; interpreting; confronting and providing feedback) were used and how effective they were in engaging the client(s) and moving the session forward.
- Review what you are doing in your music therapy sessions. Go over the techniques that have been discussed in this chapter. Which verbal, nonverbal, and musical facilitation strategies are you using; which do you feel most comfortable and confident with, and which ones do you need to improve upon? Think about ways that you can continue to increase your confidence and competence with implementation.
- Review the discussion on expressive elements. Try to think of additional expressive elements that were not mentioned. Write up a comprehensive list including the elements provided and the additional ones that you think of, and continue to add to this list as other ideas come to you.
- You are training to become a music therapist. Has reading this chapter influenced the way you think about using music? If so, write about how your thinking is changing.
- Review the discussion of Bruscia's 64 clinical techniques in combination with your list of expressive elements. Establish some structured practice strategies using these two sets of tools. For example, select three clinical techniques and three expressive elements and then work to use them in an improvisation or integrate them in a short composition. For instance, from the clinical techniques you might decide to work with the structuring technique of rhythmic grounding, the elicitation technique of making spaces, and the redirection technique of modulating, and then incorporate expressive elements of texture, ornamentation, and a third element that you have identified on your own. You may want to review Bruscia's clinical techniques in more detail as part of this assignment.
- As a follow-up to your structured practice strategy assignment, consider journaling about your experience; did this assignment provide you with greater focus and confidence in practicing improvisation and composition skills, or perhaps did you find it too limiting? Bring your thoughts about this into supervision with your clinical supervisor and/or faculty advisor; you may also want to discuss some of these strategies with your other teachers (piano, guitar, voice, percussion).

14 The Role of Music

Music has been a part of people's lives throughout history and in all cultures. Blacking (1973) stated that "musicality is a universal, species-specific characteristic" (p. 116). Thanks to modern technology, music has assumed an expanded role in society today. It helps us to integrate our lives and is a significant part of our life histories. The prevalence of music in everyday life has changed our relationship with music—creating *music habits* (Ruud, 1998).

Music is a medium that does not lend itself easily to interpretation; it has an impact at the affective and physical level. Its primitiveness can have an enormous effect on clients for whom verbal interpretation is impossible (De Backer & Van Camp, 1999). The therapist holds the responsibility to choose music for clinical intervention and may choose with a focus on the individual, systems, behaviors, attitudes, and relationships (Stige, 2002).

The role of music is at the heart of our music therapy work. The therapist's view of the role of music is based on his or her theoretical understanding. Authors in music therapy have described many roles for music in clinical treatment. Some focus primarily on the aesthetic qualities of the music and its role in connecting us to a universal order, while others give primary attention to how music connects us with others, for example, our relationships with key individuals in our lives and our music-based community bonds. Additionally, music serves to connect us to ourselves and to our place within our community and culture. Music is a resource that enriches our quality of life in these and many other ways.

Boxill (1997) speaks of the importance of music, defining music as "a basic essence of the universe and esthetic means of expression with the extraordinary power to reach the human organism on all levels—the mind, the body, the soul; it has the power to heal, to expand conscious awareness, to stimulate the full spectrum of emotion and feelings" (p. 10).

Ruud (1998) articulates the roles for music in music therapy. He believes that music plays an important role in the construction of identity. Music can serve as raw material for building value and life orientation and as a way to anchor important relationships, frame our experience in a certain time and space, and position ourselves within our culture and thus make explicit our ethnicity, gender, and class. Music also provides important *peak* or transcendental experiences that may strengthen the formation of identity and help us to feel meaning, purpose, and significance in our lives.

Aigen (2005b, 2014a) describes the importance of music in music-centered music therapy and suggests that it is the musical experience itself that is intrinsically rewarding and motivating for the client.

Engagement with music allows clients to experience the patterns of musical structure and the boundaries that it creates, along with the flow of emotional expression achieved through singing, playing, improvising, creating, and moving and listening to music. D. Aldridge (1996) views art forms, including music, dance, and visual art, as primarily concerned with the expression rather than the stimulation of emotion. For Aldridge, music and its performance are parallel processes in healthy living.

Bonde (2011) describes uses of music in a variety of formats—in music therapy, in community music settings, in medical environments—and proposes a theoretical model that he calls "health musicing." In this model, which is influenced by the work of Wilber (1996) and Ansdell (2001), Bonde presents a schema with four quadrants: (a) the development of communities and values through musicing, (b) the shaping and sharing of musical environments, (c) the professional use of music(ing) and sound(ing) to help individuals, and (d) the formation and development of identity through musicing. He emphasizes the crossover and integration of music's role in these varying applications, stressing the transformative powers of music in the lives of people.

Clair (1996, pp. 11–23) offers an overview of the many uses of music in music therapy, which can be viewed as the clinical roles of music. She suggests that music:

- Evokes a wide range of physical responses,
- Evokes related emotional responses,
- Facilitates social integration,
- Serves as form of communication,
- Communicates emotional expression,
- Evokes associations,
- Provides meaningful engagement,
- Relieves anxiety and stress,
- Structures experiences that elicit behaviors that require self-control and responsibility, and
- Offers accessible aesthetic experience.

Finally, a Massive Open Online Course (MOOC) on the topic of "How Music Can Change Your Life … and the World" (McFerran, 2016) presents six ways of understanding how music works. The questions include: How can music influence the body? How can music motivate the mind? How can music reflect the psyche? How can music foster intimacy? How can music enhance connectedness? And, How can music express culture? The MOOC includes *Voices* articles, podcasts, and interviews that explore these questions (McFerran, 2016).

Connections Through Music

To Aesthetics and Universal Order

The ability of music to produce experiences that we find difficult to put into words is an important characteristic that music shares with other aesthetic media. An aesthetic experience produced by music implies the possibility of creating a new category of experience, experiencing the world in a new way. This provides one of the most basic rationales for the use of music in therapy (Ruud, 1998). Aigen (1995) suggests that "aesthetic considerations are central to clinical music therapy process" (p. 235).

Authors writing about the role of the aesthetics of music in clinical work find that beauty itself can have a profound impact on the well-being of clients, while the patterns and structure of music provide other equally powerful means of helping clients. Kenny (1989) believes that music offers the client the opportunity to move beyond the known self. It is within the beauty of the pattern in music that the client finds safety and is able to explore. Kenny goes on to state: "The musical improvisation encourages a person to identify a pattern or way of organizing which has personal significance and meaning for the music maker" (p. 33). Aigen (1995) says, "A hallmark of aesthetic experience is a high degree of integration and meaning, aspects [of] which enhance personality development, cognitive functioning, and social interaction, which are, not incidentally, important clinical goals" (p. 237).

Thaut (2000) sees music as "a culturally based art form, an aesthetic medium, that expresses and embodies patterns, forms, and symbols associated with the structures and rules of its specific language. As such, music intrinsically communicates two meaningful contents: (a) its own structure and patterns, built by the grammatical and syntactical rules of abstract sound patterns, and, based on this, (b) the perceptual values of the listener as to the aesthetic quality, cultural meanings, and personal associations and experiences in the music" (p. 3).

Ruud (1998) espouses that "it is the poetic or aesthetic aspect of the musical communication ... that can transform the improvisation into a therapeutic tool" (p. 118). It is this participatory nature of improvisation that gives rise to a sort of meaning stemming from the dialogical nature of musical interaction.

To Others

All kinds of music around us can be seen as flexible maps of modern life worlds. These maps change when context changes, affecting how we see ourselves in relation to the world around us (Ruud, 1998). Because music is deeply embedded in our culture and world, it also plays a role in the development of culture and society and links clients to it. Music may also be seen as raw material for social life. For Ruud, it is the transformation of sound into symbol and the accompanying experience that links people into communities and societies. Social organization around aesthetic activities shows that communities are built not only by people sharing the same house, work, socioeconomic background, or neighborhood. Stige (2002) sees this connection to society in the way a therapist chooses music for practice. These choices, whether conscious or unconscious, are linked to values, traditions, and practices.

If we accept Ruud's premise that music therapy concerns social groups or society at large, improvisational music therapy is like a miniature social system. The clinical setting—the "laboratory of music therapy"—may be regarded as a place to model or construct some of the tools the client needs to become involved in a larger social system. Music therapy can be used to investigate how musical dialogue is developed and maintained through improvisational techniques (Ruud, 1998).

Music also draws us into relationships. Much of the literature focuses on the tendency for music to encourage the human system to organize. This often means that the therapist chooses music that will draw the client into a particular type of organization, as seen in rhythmic entrainment (Kenny, 1989). It is assumed that when the client sees the therapist's willingness to *entrain,* or join in his or her sound representations, the client may be encouraged to be more open to explore and entrain with the therapist's rhythms, which ideally reflect healthy patterns (pp. 36–37).

Music may assist a client in reconnecting to the world outside of him- or herself within the context of the relationship with the therapist. De Backer and Van Camp (1999) describe this phenomenon in depression and psychosis:

> When time slows down and the body no longer has the energy to free itself from gravitation—as in depression—or when time has stopped and the subject is excluded from a symbolically shared experience—as in psychosis— it is often solely music which succeeds in making a connection between the concrete untranslatable musical sound and rhythm and the extinguished tempo of the patient. As a child who is carried and contained by the musical exchange with his/her mother during the first period of life, a depressive or psychotic patient can only connect again with life through those same physical and affective exchanges. (p. 16)

To Self

Music can connect one's identity to one's expression. Music therapists may use musical genres that are associated with cultural or societal issues with parallels to a client's personal issues (Ruud, 1998).

Stige (2002) connects musical activities—including listening, playing, creating, performing, interpreting, and reflecting—to artifacts—such as instruments, songs, words, and metaphors used in the music therapy process—and argues that cultural artifacts are important in a person's development of self and identity. Thus, a person's sense of self and agency is constituted through internalization and creative use of cultural artifacts in social contexts. From Stige's point of view, each musical experience is connected to the self and to society.

Singing can help clients to access and express feelings while also providing them with an experience that is creative and often pleasurable. Singing is a way to melt walls—walls that were constructed initially to protect the vulnerable child or adolescent but are no longer necessary, that now serve only to separate the individual from the vitality of the authentic self trapped within and that isolate a person from the outer world and meaningful connections with others (Austin, 1999). When vocal improvisation is used, it may serve to (a) establish trust, (b) comfort and soothe, (c) access unconscious memories and/or associations, (d) work through resistance to feelings, (e) deepen feelings, and (f) help a client who has dissociated move gently back into his or her body and become more emotionally present (Austin, 1999).

Austin (2008) describes specific vocal techniques that can help connect the client to him- or herself. Mirroring is especially useful when a client needs support in finding his or her own voice. This musical reflection provides encouragement and can assist in strengthening the client's sense of self. Clients often report that the experience of being heard and answered in the music results in a feeling of recognition and validation. Grounding occurs when the therapist sings the root of the chords, thereby providing a base for the client's improvisation. The client can then explore musically and return home for refueling. When singing a cappella or with nonharmonic instruments, the therapist can hold one note and create a dronelike effect over which the client can improvise.

Another important aspect of connecting with the self is the choice of instruments used to make music, as this is one of many elements in the search for one's own musical expression. Additionally, the client's choice of instrument reveals a lot about the unconscious symbolic meaning that he or she attaches to the instrument. Of course, the symbolic meaning of instruments can have a variety of possible interpretations, all of which are subjective. Certainly, the choice of instrument is influenced by the previous experience and cultural background of the patient (De Backer & Van Camp, 1999).

Improvisation may be a good metaphor for understanding the individual. We often start from scratch, from some preliminary ideas. Although we may have some broader notions of where we want to go, we can never be sure of either the route to follow or the final goal. When improvising with another person, the music we make is influenced by others in a circular manner—as are the plans that we make for life. In the process, we may find a new tempo, transpose, take risks, and meet crises involving a possible breakdown in the improvisation—much as in life. Through the process of improvisation, we may come up with a product in a certain style and thus create our own piece of musical identity, much as our personal identity is improvised and narrated (Ruud, 1998).

Involvement with music can produce a strong, flexible, and differentiated identity and is a potential resource for obtaining a better quality of life (Ruud, 1998). Music may be a source of social enrichment and may stimulate communication and intellectual curiosity, to name only a few. If being involved in music generally strengthens our sense of identity and if having a strong and differentiated sense of identity is connected to a higher quality of life, then it follows that music contributes to health in general (Ruud, 1998).

Using Connections Through Music

In discussing the role of music in music therapy, Bruscia (1987, pp. 8–9, 503–504; 2014, pp. 45–46) makes a distinction between music *as* therapy and music *in* therapy. When the client's relationship to the music is primary, music is used *as* therapy. When the client's relationship to the therapist is primary, music is used *in* therapy. More recently, the idea of music *as* therapy has been further explored and explained by Aigen (2005b, 2014a) and is now widely referred to as "music-centered music therapy." Regardless of which choice is made for a specific client, music therapy is distinguished by heavy reliance on musical experience as the agent, context, or catalyst for the therapeutic experience. Thus, it becomes imperative for the music therapist to understand various dimensions of musical experience and how they become therapeutic in nature. Music offers therapeutic benefits from both its active and receptive qualities. When therapy is active, the client is involved in performing, improvising, or creating music. When therapy is receptive, the client listens, takes in, or receives the music itself.

Whether your clinical work involves music *as* therapy or music *in* therapy, it is necessary to develop the music skills that will allow you to design musical experiences that lead toward client goals. The next section explores ways in which these musical experiences can be implemented.

Developing Clinical Musicianship

As you develop a base of knowledge about various client populations, it will become increasingly apparent that you will need to develop a broad range of musical awareness and skills and a diverse repertoire. Each population and every individual served demands different music and music experiences. Perhaps the best place to begin is to take time to examine your own relationship with music, your musical preferences and dislikes, your musical strengths and needs, and your use of music in your personal life. Several articles that can help you with this exploration include "How Do We Nurture Ourselves?" (Amir, 2001a), "Sometimes, It Is Our Task to Find Out How Much Music We Can Still Make with What We Have Left" (Amir, 2001b), "Music and Symbols" (Deschênes, 1995), and "The Transformative Power of Music in Our Lives: A Personal Perspective" (Hesser, 2001).

When working with instruments, keep in mind that choice plays an important role. The instrument selection of the music therapist immediately reveals something about the possibilities and the limitation in his or her practice. It also indicates how he or she views music as a medium, observes the client, and so on (De Backer & Van Camp, 1999).

We will consider the development of clinical musicianship as it applies to the four main methods in music therapy—improvising, re-creating, compositional, and receptive experiences (Bruscia, 2014b). As you consider them this time, think about them in personal terms, as they apply to you. This is a step in expanding your musical awareness.

Improvising Experiences

For the client, the clinical outcomes of improvising experiences may include the development of nonverbal communication skills, the exploration of self in relation to others, the creation of an outlet for self-expression, and experimentation within structure (Bruscia, 2014b). The value of developing your own improvisation skills outside of the therapy setting cannot be overstated—in a therapy session, a music therapist must be able to experiment within structure each time instantaneous revisions must be made to the existing session plan. Appreciate that improvisation is far more than just a way of playing music—it is a basic skill in the therapist's interaction with the client.

Discussing piano improvisation in a purely musical sense, Chase (1974) said:

> Free improvisation is a pleasure that has been denied to too many musicians. It is often one of the first things that will be discouraged in a child. This denial is usually based on the idea that there is a prescribed and "correct" way to use the piano, and unless the child has mastered that, she has no right to use her own ideas. If a child is not intimidated at a young age, she can enjoy discovering all kinds of sound patterns on an instrument. She can develop a tremendous sense of freedom with the instrument and with her own expressiveness. It will give her a sense of friendship and intimacy with the instrument that can be acquired in no other way. (p. 67)

Chase (1974) goes on to state:

> Once you have discovered the pleasure of this free experimentation, enjoy it and don't censor or judge yourself because you will only lock up your creativity again. If you do not like what you hear, do not let yourself interfere with the process. Eventually, when you stop thinking and evaluating and can just let it happen, you will find that you have reopened an avenue for more interesting creations to come to the fore. (pp. 70–71)

The beginning stages of developing improvisation skills can be intimidating. Start with a simple structure and call on your own creative instinct. Wigram (2004) provides step-by-step guidance and resources for the development of improvisation skills in a personal manner yet for clinical application.

Trust—in yourself and in the music—is critical. Jordan (1999) states "Music making is constructed of correct notes, correct rhythms, dynamics, and articulation. But the mortar of music is human trust (of self and others)" (p. 11). He also says "Knowledge and trust of self is necessary for music making to take place. An ability to 'just be' is paramount" (p. 10). This idea, to just be, holds tremendous importance in music and in therapy. Maslow (1999) discusses this extensively in his descriptions of humanistic psychology and the concept of moving to higher levels of self-actualization. As part of this growth, there is an emphasis on ways of observing the world around us. Maslow characterizes this as a childlike sense of the world that is open to experience and is spontaneous and expressive. This is natural in children and is found in self-actualizing, creative persons. Maslow postulates that these qualities are either retained from childhood or regained in those who are able to express themselves without fear of ridicule. He believes this to be a fundamental, inherent characteristic of human nature. As you work on your improvisatory skills, allow yourself to regain this way of knowing and being with music.

Re-creative Experiences

For the client, the clinical outcomes of re-creative experiences may include the development of interpretive skills; the improvement of interactive and group skills; and the enhancement of sensorimotor, attention, and memory skills. These experiences include singing, playing, or performing precomposed music, engaging in musical games and musical shows, and conducting a group in music-making (Bruscia, 2014b).

The therapist must develop the ability to design and implement these musical experiences in order to engage the client and facilitate participation that addresses the client's goals. This includes skill in sequencing tasks, giving clear directions, providing cues and assistance, and assessing the experience and making necessary adjustments to maximize successful music-making. In order to develop these skills, it may be useful to note the steps involved when you are engaged in a re-creative musical experience in a class or other musical group. Another useful exercise blends improvising with re-creating, or incorporates a transitional process. Pay close attention when you are improvising freely; when you find that you have created a powerful pattern (harmonic, rhythmic, or melodic in nature), immediately attempt to re-create it. Not only can this help you improve your aural attention, it can lay the groundwork for moving you into practical composing experiences, as described below. Practice these skills whenever you have the opportunity.

Compositional Experiences

For the client, the clinical outcomes of compositional experiences may include the development of organizational and planning skills; the improvement of the ability to document and communicate inner experiences; the refinement of the ability to sequence, integrate, and synthesize parts into wholes; and the promotion of decision-making skills (Bruscia, 2014b).

Here, as with improvising, you must allow the spontaneous, creative nature you were born with to rise to the surface. Composing may have some specific musical rules, but most important is that you learn to compose freely in order to prepare yourself to assist others in learning to compose creatively. You should also work toward blending aspects of composing with improvising and re-creating experiences, as this can be an effective strategy for thematic development in clinical music.

Receptive Experiences

The clinical outcomes of receptive experiences for the client may include stimulation or relaxation; evoking affective states, imagery, and fantasies; facilitating memory and reminiscence; and stimulating peak and spiritual experiences (Bruscia, 2014b). When therapy involves listening to music, it is essential to consider whether the music has the aesthetic qualities needed to motivate the client to engage in the therapeutic process, as well as whether it has the physical and psychological qualities needed to induce positive changes (Bruscia, 2014b). In other words, the music selected for receptive experiences should have qualities that make it worth using. The musical knowledge that music therapy students acquire through their training provides the basis for selecting music with the aesthetic, physical, and psychological qualities that are desired.

Consider keeping a *personal listening journal,* in which you can write about the following:

- When do you listen to music?
- Where do you listen to music?
- What music do you listen to?
- What purposes/outcomes do you hope to accomplish?

- What other sorts of activities or tasks do you engage in while listening to music?
- Do you share music listening experiences with others? If so, with whom and why?

Chase (1974) discusses the value of recording your own playing, suggesting that it is "an excellent source for self-teaching. It reflects your playing back to yourself, for in listening to the recording, the discrepancies between your wishful listening and your playing will be revealed" (p. 38). In undertaking this process, you allow yourself the luxury of capturing all the nuances of your increasing personal and clinical musicianship and the opportunity to identify themes for future development.

Summary

This chapter has offered an overview of several theories about the role of music in music therapy, framed within the understanding that music has three broad purposes, all related to connection. First, music may be a means to connect us to something greater than the material world—the aesthetic or universal order. Second, music may also connect us to the world around us through relationships with cultures, groups, or individuals. Third, music offers us avenues to connect more deeply to ourselves and to explore our inner world. As the therapist, you must become fluid in your ability to work in each of these realms. This chapter offers suggestions for exploring and developing your relationship with and skills in using music. Use the assignments to access your own creativity and to develop the skills for providing therapeutic musical experiences to your clients.

Assignments—The Role of Music

These assignments will help you to examine, understand, and develop your understanding of the role of music:

- Over the course of 1 week, keep a *personal listening journal,* as described above. Include the following:
  - When are you listening to music?
  - Where are you listening to music?
  - What music are you listening to?
  - What purposes/outcomes are you hoping to accomplish? (Your purpose may be as simple as enjoyment.)
  - What other sorts of activities or tasks are you engaging in while listening to music?
  - Are you sharing music listening experiences with others? If so, with whom and why? If not, why do you this is the case?
- Consider the four main experiences in music therapy (improvising, re-creative, compositional, and receptive) as described by Bruscia (2014b), but this time, think about them in personal terms. Do a self-assessment that includes: (a) your personal experiences with each type of experience; (b) your experiences as a beginning music therapist with each type of experience; and (c) what you can do to become more familiar with and comfortable using each type of experience.
- Consider the connections between improvising, re-creative, compositional, and receptive experiences. Practice the following exercise. You can do this on any instrument, but particularly try to create opportunities to explore this with the four

primary clinical instruments of piano, guitar, voice, and percussion.

○ Begin with a simple structure within which you can improvise.

○ As you continue to develop your theme, notice how you naturally engage in re-creating it, exploring different colorations in it each time you explore it.

○ Experiment with emerging themes over a series of playing times or days, and notice how it takes on a sense of structure so that you can utilize it at will (or as a situation in therapy might dictate); at this point, notate it.

○ Record it for your own review to uncover its strengths and potentials, or use it in a setting in which you may not have access to the necessary equipment and instruments, ultimately providing a listening experience for your clients.

○ Write about this experience.

• Look again at the second assignment listed above. For each type of musical experience (improvising, re-creative, compositional, and receptive), evaluate how your personal experiences and your experiences as a beginning music therapist might be changing over time. What have you done to become more familiar with and comfortable using each type of experience? Write out a plan to develop the areas in which you would like to make greater progress.

15 Working with Groups

Many music therapy sessions are provided in a group format. There are a number of reasons for this. Some of them are economic—it is less expensive to treat people in groups, and one music therapist can see more people when they are seen together. But there are reasons unrelated to economics why music therapy is done in groups. The most important reason for treating people in groups is that, since we lead much of our lives in social situations, many of the problems that we encounter occur in social situations. So what better way to work on problems than in the same arena in which we have the problems?

Of course, the other members of a music therapy group are probably not the people with whom a client has a problem in *real life.* (An exception to this would be in a family music therapy group, which typically includes some of the people with whom real problems are encountered.) Herein lies one of the most potent reasons that groups can be effective: They create the safety and support necessary to help clients work through problems they encounter outside of the group, thus helping them to become healthier and more effective in real life. Many music therapy groups are set up to do this.

Working with groups of a similar chronological age, such as we find in most schools, has the benefit of presenting similar developmental challenges, which can help the music therapist to plan and work more effectively. In some special education settings, the level of functioning is a primary consideration, although age is also taken into account.

Various institutional settings may also consider age when placing people in groups. In many inpatient and outpatient treatment settings for people with emotional difficulties, a person's age is a primary consideration in the program to which he or she is admitted. It is quite usual to have one treatment facility or unit for adolescents, one for adults, and one for older adults. We are all familiar with nursing homes, where most people are older, although some younger people requiring extensive care (such as survivors of severe traumatic brain injury) may be admitted. As with children in schools, age grouping brings people of similar sociocultural backgrounds together, while clients of similar ages are also more likely to be working on similar life tasks, for example, groups of older adults dealing with aging and loss.

Sometimes people who function at similar levels are placed together. The consideration may be what they are able to do or their developmental level. Sometimes, for instance, people who need a high level of care stay in one part of a facility, while those who need less intensive care are placed in another part.

In some settings, age and level of functioning are not the determining factors; people are placed together when they have similar needs or characteristics. In schools, again, it is not unusual for children with emotional difficulties to be placed together, those with communication problems to be placed together, those with intellectual deficits to be placed together, and so forth. (Such homogenous placement has decreased markedly in recent years with the belief that it is better for children to be educated with children who are not classified as having problems—in other words, in the mainstream or, as it is referred to most often, in an inclusion setting.) Similarly, rehabilitation centers will often place people with spinal cord injuries in one area and those with head injuries in another area. Finally, adults with addictions or with emotional problems are often placed together. Even though people placed in groups have similar characteristics, it is important to remember that within those groupings there will be different needs and levels of functioning. Maslow (1999) devotes attention to this issue, saying:

> To place a person in a system takes less energy than to know him in his own right, since in the former instance, all that has to be perceived is that one abstracted characteristic which indicates his belongingness in a class. ... What is stressed in rubricizing is the category in which the person belongs, of which he is a sample, not the person as such—similarities rather than differences. (p. 141)

Two points should be made as we discuss separating people by age, level of functioning, and type of problem. The first is that all labels are potentially damaging and must be used with great care. When we say that one person is "high-functioning" while another is "low-functioning," we are using a label that may have a negative connotation and lead to results that we did not intend. We must, therefore, use labels for the purpose for which they are intended but be very careful not to rely too much on them. The second point is that more than one category or label can be applied to all of us. If people are placed in categories by labels, it is important to realize that such placement will be only partly accurate. A child placed in a group because of emotional difficulties, for instance, may also have communication difficulties or be very gifted. Always strive to remember that clients are complex individuals and not their labels or diagnoses.

Music therapists have addressed music therapy in groups in a number of books and other writings. Books include *Group Analytic Music Therapy* by Ahonen-Eerikäinen (2007); *Music Therapy: Group Vignettes* by Borczon (1997); *Music Therapy and Group Work: Sound Company* by Davies and Richards (2002); *Group Music Therapy: A Group Analytic Approach* by Davies, Richards, and Barwick (2014); *Music Therapy Improvisation for Groups: Essential Leadership Competencies* by Gardstrom (2007); *Music Therapy Groupwork with Special Needs Children* (Goodman, 2007); and *Groups in Music: Strategies From Music Therapy* by Pavlicevic (2003).

Forming Music Therapy Groups

People are often assigned to a music therapy group based on their participation in other groups. For example, children who share a classroom for their educational activities may be assigned to music therapy together or a group of clients with psychiatric difficulties may have music therapy scheduled at a particular time in their day. For reasons we've already discussed, this can be a very effective division. An additional benefit is that the clients will already know each other and may, as a result, be more comfortable working together.

Instead of grouping by age and characteristics, a music therapist may have the freedom to identify people to include in a music therapy group. In such a situation, the music therapist decides the basis for the grouping, then assesses the potential group members (often in consultation with others who work with them) to determine group membership. This allows people to be grouped for various reasons—perhaps because they are dealing with similar issues or function at similar levels.

Other music therapy groups are formed based on who expresses an interest in music or music therapy. This is how groups are often formed in treatment facilities for adults with emotional difficulties and in nursing homes and other facilities for older adults. The advantage of this method is that those who attend music therapy do so by choice.

Music therapists who work in community settings are likely to work with configurations of people who are already part of a group. One of the advantages here is that working with people in their natural environment enriches and builds on their community ties. Although music therapists have worked in community settings for many years, Community Music Therapy (Pavlicevic & Ansdell, 2004; Stige, 2002; Stige & Aarø, 2012; Stige, Ansdell, Elefant, & Pavlicevic, 2010) is defining, developing, and popularizing this work and helping music therapists to understand their role and the role of music therapy in the community.

Short-Term Treatment

Another consideration in forming music therapy groups is whether the setting is long- or short-term. This is not normally an issue in school settings for children, since most schools' placements are for at least a year, although it may be in other treatment settings for children. It is not generally an issue in nursing home placements or some other placements for older adults, since these tend to be long-term placements. In rehabilitation, medical, and mental health settings, though, many clients will be in the treatment facility for very short periods of time. Due to philosophical, insurance, and other reasons, some clients may stay only a day or two, while even those whose stays are relatively lengthy may be in treatment for only three or four weeks. The philosophical reason for shorter stays is the belief that people are better off living in their normal environment and receiving ongoing treatment there than living in an institution. The insurance reason is that, with attempts being made to cut health care costs, institutional stays are closely monitored and limited. The result of these shorter stays in certain treatment settings is that clients are seen only briefly in music therapy.

Music therapy can be tailored for people with short-term stays. Music therapists can often schedule clients more times per week than they might if the clients were there longer. In a single week, for instance, music therapy might meet three or five times, thus accomplishing goals in a more compact form. The goals of short-term treatment may be quite different from goals in long-term treatment, often focusing on crisis intervention, restoration of functioning, and helping clients access resources in the community for further treatment and support.

Methods and expectations must also be adapted to short-term treatment. What is to be accomplished must be accomplished more quickly, at times within a single session. This changes much of the process of therapy, with assessment needing to occur very quickly within the session, methods being easily comprehensible, and evaluation occurring on an ongoing basis.

Music therapists working in short-term settings become skillful at adapting to new clients. With turnover occurring so quickly, people often attend the music therapy session without the therapist being acquainted with their problems, history, and interests, all of which would be available in a long-term setting. Students who work in short-term treatment settings, often spending only a few hours or days at the facility, find special challenges in working with clients about whom they have limited previous knowledge. In these settings, it becomes imperative for the student to maintain ongoing communication with the on-site supervisor in order to provide music therapy experiences that are meaningful and appropriate for the clients.

Short-term group work may also be applied in community settings and be offered to people in a variety of situations. Short-term groups have been offered to address needs of parents of children with special needs (Nicholson, Berthelsen, Abad, Williams, & Bradley, 2008), of persons who have experienced natural disasters (McFerran & Teggelove, 2011), of those who have experienced trauma that has led to posttraumatic stress disorder (Borczon, 1997, Chapter 10), and of those with intellectual disabilities who have been deinstitutionalized (in this case, through a weekend cultural festival) (Stige, Ansdell, Elefant, & Pavlicevic, 2010, Chapters 9, 10).

Level of Structure

Music therapy groups may be organized in various ways. To clarify some of the differences, it can be helpful to view music therapy groups according to the level of structure and extent of the direction provided by the therapist. A leader who uses a *directive* style leads (or directs) the group, establishing the type of music therapy experience and leading group members through the planned activity. One who uses a *nondirective* style provides little direction to the group but allows and encourages the direction to emerge from the group itself.

Although it can be useful to consider group leadership in terms of how directive or nondirective it is, there are also difficulties with doing this. One is that many groups include elements of both leadership styles. Another is that sometimes a person uses elements of one style on one occasion and the other style on another, making it impossible to classify the leadership style as directive or nondirective.

Groups with leaders who use a directive style of leadership will often fall into the categories of activity therapy (Wheeler, 1983) or supportive, activities-oriented music therapy (Unkefer & Thaut, 2002). It can be challenging to discern which levels of structure may be needed for any particular group on any particular day, and flexibility on the part of the therapist is crucial. Keep in mind the various theoretical models that were previously described.

Much of the literature on working with older adults refers to groups with directive leadership. Clair and Memmott (2008), citing literature indicating that social activity, personal control, and opportunities to increase their knowledge and skills are helpful in promoting a sense of well-being in older adults, recommends activities that ...

> (1) promote social interaction with others, (2) offer opportunities to make decisions and manage choices, (3) present occasions to learn or relearn information or skills, and (4) provide opportunities to discover novel ways to use personal resources (p. 37).

Clair goes on to suggest that participation in music offers all of these and more. These goals and ways of thinking about therapy lend themselves to an activity therapy style of working. Chavin (1991), writing about the use of music to reach people with dementia, also cites goals and ways of working within an activity therapy approach to music therapy. Other descriptions of the use of music therapy with people with dementia (e.g., Brotons & Marti, 2003; Ledger & Baker, 2007) also appear to utilize a directive leadership style.

Another example of a group in which the music therapist took a directive role in leadership is by M. Cassity (1976), who studied the influence on the peer acceptance, group cohesiveness, and interpersonal relationships of a music therapy group in which clients with psychiatric difficulties learned to play the guitar. The therapist, who was teaching participants to play the guitar, no doubt used a directive leadership style.

While some groups can benefit from planned activities and strong guidance, keep in mind that, with a directive style, the group comes to depend upon the therapist to keep the group going and make group decisions. If the therapist is trying to get group members to take increasing responsibility for what occurs in the group, a less directive approach should be used. Although this can occur in many music therapy contexts, songwriting could provide a good example of how it would work. Although it was not part of their study, the songwriting protocol developed by Tamplin, Baker, Macdonald, Roddy, and Rickard (2016) helps to illustrate this point. They present a 12-session songwriting protocol to promote integration of self-concept in people with acquired neurological injuries. The first four sessions are spent composing a song about the past; the next four, about the present; and the final four, about the future. Their protocol repeats itself for each new composition—in other words, after each sequence of four sessions. A way that the same protocol could be used—but with decreasing directiveness by the therapist and thus more responsibility or control by the client—would be for the music therapist to intentionally provide less guidance in each successive phase, although, of course, being available to contribute more if necessary. We could see that, by doing this, clients would gradually assume more responsibility for the development of the song.

Many music therapy groups follow procedures planned by the leader or facilitator, with the purpose of this sequence being to elicit musical and nonmusical responses from the group members. The procedures are intended to facilitate the work of the group. This style of group leadership is not as directive as those described above, in that the leader does not typically direct everything. However, it may be quite directive in how the group is structured, leading the group to be a combination of directive and nondirective. The groups described in the next paragraphs are examples of this type of group, where several experiences are structured to assist the group members in working on their goals.

Plach (1980) uses this format, incorporating a sequence of experiences, in *The Creative Use of Music in Group Therapy* when he describes a group in which a song is used to stimulate discussion, personal work, or group process.

The group vignettes described by Borczon (1997) in *Music Therapy: Group Vignettes* include elements of this format, with the musical activity providing a focus for the later development of the group. Borczon describes a number of vignettes, which give a sense of the richness of material that can be a part of a music therapy group. He also makes the point that group sessions are composed of an opening, a main portion (the one of which most writers speak), and a closing. Treder-Wolff (1990) describes the benefits of music therapy experiences, particularly the use of popular songs and lyric analysis, in addictions treatment group work. She emphasizes the importance of how these experiences can support clients in learning about their disease, breaking down defensiveness and denial, recognizing and accepting the illness, and taking responsibility for recovery and continuing participation in treatment in order to prevent relapse. She describes an approach that starts with the therapist being directive and gradually becoming somewhat nondirective, having the group take on increasing responsibility for the work.

Many music therapy groups are based on improvisation. As described by Dvorkin (1998), these groups utilize music improvisation and clients' reactions to the improvisation. The therapist in these groups has an important role in facilitating the improvisation and verbal processing of the experience (when that occurs). Gardstrom (2007) offers specific exercises for students to develop skills in leading and processing group improvisation. Facilitators of groups that utilize improvisation may be directive or nondirective or use elements of both. Analytical Music Therapy (Priestley, 1975, 1994) may also use group improvisation and may employ a less directive approach.

A leaderless group is the most nondirective type of group experience. Although this is not a typical music therapy format, it is theoretically possible. Even in a leaderless group, leaders tend to emerge in order to help the group function.

Stages of Development

Groups evolve through various stages over time. These stages have been identified in various ways but generally include the same basic sequence. The four stages, as identified by Corey, Corey, Callanan, and Russell (2014), are the initial stage, the transition stage, the working stage, and the ending stage.

During the *initial stage,* trust is developing and members (as well as the leader) are dealing with anxiety over what the group will entail. Members wonder how to get involved, may be concerned about outcomes, and begin developing roles, forming power structures, and testing the leader and other members. During the *transition stage,* group members learn to recognize and deal with anxiety, resistance, and conflict. Members must learn to monitor their feelings and reactions and to express them. The leader at this stage must develop interventions that help a group to become a cohesive unit. During the *working stage,* the work of the group, or the purpose for which it has been formed, is accomplished. Characteristics of this stage are that members are usually eager to initiate work or to bring up themes and are willing to interact with one another, including having confrontations. This stage is characterized by a here-and-now focus. Members can usually identify their goals and concerns and take responsibility for them. Group cohesion increases during this stage. Termination occurs during the *ending stage.* During this time, members complete any unfinished business and prepare for the ending of the group. They also make plans to continue to deal with issues and receive support when the group no longer exists.

The Corey, Corey, Callanan, and Russell (2014) model deals with termination as an important part of therapy. This significant phase of the therapy process is often neglected but is important and should be given consideration. McGuire and Smeltekop (1994a, 1994b) reviewed the literature on termination of therapy and developed a model that is appropriate for termination in both group and individual music therapy. It includes the following sequence: (a) termination announcement, (b) review and evaluation, (c) expression of feelings, (d) projections into the future, and (e) saying good-bye. Music therapy students are encouraged to pay attention to this stage, which can sometimes be difficult to deal with because of our own feelings, as well as those of our clients, about ending therapy. It is precisely because of these feelings that the termination of therapy should be acknowledged and addressed.

Stages of music therapy groups have been dealt with only occasionally in the music therapy literature. Hibben's (1991) group followed a progression similar to the one above. She describes the stages of development of a group of 6- through 8-year-old children with attention deficit hyperactivity disorder, utilizing three stages of group development posited by Garland, Jones, and Kolodny (1976). The group began in the *pre-affiliation stage,* during which children were acting as individuals but not yet functioning as a group. When they moved into the *power and control stage,* they began to jockey for positions in the group; during this stage, the therapist gave control to the children as much as possible. In the third stage, the *intimacy stage,* the children began using the group to practice new behaviors. During this latter stage, "the therapist's aim was to move the children to take more responsibility for the group activities, to urge them to make the rules, to be the leaders, and to share their intimate selves" (Hibben, p. 183). Hibben's description of group process and stages is significant in that it follows the typical progression described in the literature. This occurred because she was nondirective enough to allow the group to develop as it needed to and also aware enough of group development that she allowed and facilitated the needs of the members at each stage.

James and Freed (1989) proposed a five-stage model to develop group cohesion in music therapy:

- Stage 1: Goal-setting activities,
- Stage 2: Individual/parallel activities,
- Stage 3: Cooperative group activities,
- Stage 4: Self-disclosure activities,
- Stage 5: Group problem-solving activities.

Their model is different from the others, in that they appear to be providing a directive approach to moving the group through stages rather than facilitating the group's own movement through the stages. Although there is no report of this model having been tested, it might prove useful for music therapists who work in a structured manner to help their groups move through various stages of group development.

Therapeutic Factors

Yalom (1985, Chapters 1–4) describes the primary factors that make the group experience therapeutic. The factors are listed below, with brief explanations of each.

1) *Instillation of hope:* Because people in a therapy group are at different points in the process of becoming healthy, a new member (or one who is struggling) can often be encouraged by seeing the progress that others have made.

2) *Universality:* People often assume that they are the only person who has a particular problem or trait; learning that others have similar concerns can be helpful.

3) *Imparting of information:* This includes didactic information about the illness or resources for assistance or information and advice that is often given by other group members.

4) *Altruism:* People are able to help others in a therapy group and may benefit by being helpful.

5) *The corrective recapitulation of the primary family group:* Many people have had problems in their primary family group, and the therapy group offers an opportunity to reenact some of these experiences and relationships in a healthier manner.

6) *Development of socializing techniques:* The social learning that occurs in therapy groups can take place at many levels, allowing people to benefit at their level of need.

7) *Imitative behavior:* Group members model their behavior after the behaviors of both the therapist and other clients.

8) *Interpersonal learning:* The relationships that develop through the therapy group, the emotional experiences that are often a part of the group experience, and the fact that the group can serve as a social microcosm all lead to unique opportunities for social learning.

9) *Group cohesiveness:* The cohesiveness of the group influences and motivates members to be accepted by others in the group, leading to behaviors and emotions that are acceptable within the group culture.

10) *Catharsis:* The opportunity to experience intense feelings in a supportive environment and to learn to express them, and for this expression to be acceptable, can be valuable.

11) *Existential factors:* These include gaining awareness that life is sometimes unjust, facing issues of life and death, and recognizing that pain is a part of life.

These factors describe qualities that might exist as a part of the group process or as a characteristic of the therapist's approach to the clients. For example, instillation of hope may be the result of interaction between and among group members or may come from the approach and attitude of the therapist.

These are important factors. Some may be more be relevant to groups with relatively nondirective leaders than to groups where the leader takes a very directive role. Some of the factors, though, apply to all groups.

Principles of Working with Groups

Some elements of group work are similar to individual work, while others are quite different. One thing that students often find confusing is that, although the group will have group goals, it is also necessary to work toward the goals of individuals within the group. Most of the primary goals will usually be similar for the majority of the members, but the therapist must also be aware of individual goals, since it is individuals who come to the group for help. Therapists have various ways of determining and documenting these individual goals along with the group goals.

Plach (1980) suggests the following guidelines for planning and implementing music in group therapy:

1) The chosen activity should be appropriately in tune with individual symptomotology [sic], individual and group needs, and within whatever conceptual, integrative, or physical limitations are existent within the group.
2) Music chosen for a session must take into consideration the cultural and age factors existent within the group.
3) The amount of structure contained in the activity is contingent upon the level of functioning of the group and its individual members.
4) The level of participation by the leader in the music activity is determined by what the group needs to experience the activity to its fullest potential.
5) All individual and group responses to a music activity are valid responses.
6) Whenever appropriate, communicate immediate observations of behavior in the music activity to the group and/or individuals in the group.
7) Whenever appropriate, refer back to the initial activity and group or individual responses to the activity.
8) Whenever appropriate, explore within the group ways of integrating newfound insights, behaviors, or skills into situations outside of the group. (p. 12)

Assignments—Working with Groups

Use these assignments to develop your understanding of working with groups:

- In your current group practicum, how was the group formed? What or who determined who would be a member of the group? If you do not already know this, speak with the music therapist who is responsible for the group to explore the answers.

- Is the therapist leading the group, or are you using a directive style, a combination of directive and nondirective, or a nondirective style? Give your reasons for labeling the style as you have.
- Examine the group stages of your group using several of the frameworks outlined in the chapter. Specifically, place it in the initial stage, the transition stage, the working stage, and the ending stage (Corey, Corey, Callanan, and Russell); you may use the stages described by Hibben if they seem to fit your group better. Then look at the group according to the stages suggested by James and Freed.
- Go through the guidelines described by Plach and speak of how you have or have not followed each in the group. If appropriate, look at the effects of following or not following each guideline.
- If appropriate to your group, describe the therapeutic factors (as described by Yalom) as they apply.

16 Working with Individuals

Music therapy can be done individually as well as in groups. The decision to assign a client to a group treatment setting or an individual setting is based on a number of factors. First, consider which setting will most effectively address the client's goals. Second, think about the kinds of interventions you plan to use and how the structure of an individual setting will contribute to those interventions as compared with the structure of a group. Most important, keep in mind the disposition of the client—will he or she function better with individual attention, or will the interaction and dynamics of a group setting be more conducive to growth?

Bruscia (1987) reports that certain models of improvisational music therapy employ only an individual or only a group format, whereas other models implement the two formats at different stages of therapeutic growth, and still others include clients in both individual and group settings simultaneously. Whether in an individual or group setting, much of what happens in therapy is similar. However, there are also important differences to consider when making the choice of individual or group sessions. This chapter examines these considerations, focusing on the use of music therapy with individuals.

Individual music therapy is indicated when a person has needs that can be worked through more easily or more effectively in an individual setting. These may be emotional needs; for example, a person is too emotionally distressed over a major life change to attend a group right away. In this case, individual work can build rapport and decrease the client's distress, leading to participation in groups. In other cases, a person may require individual therapy prior to beginning group music therapy—perhaps a child's behavior is too disturbed to allow participation in a group, but after a period of individual music therapy, he or she is ready to join a group. Sometimes, it is simply the case that the client cannot leave his or her room and thus must be treated there.

There are times when it may be useful for a person to be seen in both individual and group music therapy. In these cases, the therapist should consider whether to introduce the client to an existing group or to develop a new group. Frequently, the familiarity of certain experiences in individual therapy (e.g., certain songs for greetings and good-byes, the use of dependable prompt sequences, the learning of precomposed instrumental pieces) can allow clients to feel a sense of community with other group members, even in their first group session.

Determining whether a client should be placed in individual or group music therapy is one of the most important decisions a therapist makes. As a student music therapist, you may not have the luxury or responsibility of making these determinations, but you should certainly be sensitive to the fact that a particular client may progress at a faster or slower rate depending on the therapeutic format used. "Individual or one-to-one sessions are most appropriate: when the client is too withdrawn or aggressive for working with other clients; when a relationship with the therapist is a priority for treatment; and when the client needs privacy to work through problems" (Bruscia 1987, p. 510).

Therapists often find that individual therapy greatly increases the level of participation for both the client and therapist. Additionally, it is often the case that the role assumed by the music in the individual session takes on much greater importance, since there is less opportunity for social conversation to occur as it naturally does in group therapy.

It is important for the therapist to consider adaptations to his or her style of leading when working in individual therapy. In individual therapy, some clients may feel that there is a great deal of pressure to perform or produce, as he or she is the only person there. Others may welcome the opportunity for the individualized support and guidance; for them, it is a freeing experience, allowing greater opportunities for exploration and creativity.

Working with clients in individual sessions also raises the issue of establishing appropriate boundaries, which are necessary for developing a successful therapeutic relationship. Therapists must remember that the client is a client, not a friend. The client is in therapy to address specific problems, work toward goals, and develop the skills to live more effectively in daily life. Therapists must use caution when revealing personal information to clients, must not accept valuable gifts from clients, and must not have contact with clients beyond the scope of the therapeutic relationship. The AMTA *Code of Ethics* (American Music Therapy Association, 2014a) outlines important boundaries for client–therapist relationships and serves as a guide for music therapists. Dileo (2000) provides extensive guidance regarding ethical practice in music therapy, as well.

In some clinical settings, a student music therapist may be assigned to work with an individual early in the experience. This may be done so that the student can focus on the needs of just one client before trying to accommodate the needs of an entire group. Summer (2001) discusses supervising students working with individuals in a first practicum. Although her chapter is aimed at supervisors, it might provide students with some insights into clinical work with individuals.

Many examples of individual music therapy are found in the music therapy literature. Some collections of case studies, most of which are with individuals and most of which are edited books, include the following: Aigen's *Paths of Development in Nordoff-Robbins Music Therapy* (1998), Bruscia's *Case Studies in Music Therapy* (1991), Hadley's *Psychodynamic Music Therapy* (2003), Hibben's *Inside Music Therapy: Client Experiences* (1999), and Meadows's *Developments in Music Therapy Practice: Case Study Perspectives* (2011).

In addition, Bruscia (see www.barcelonapublishers.com) has compiled a number of collections of case studies, all titles beginning with *"Case Examples of ..."*. These collections provide rich examples of individual music therapy; many other case studies are found throughout the literature.

Some of the same considerations that are found in working with groups also apply to individuals. One of these, level of structure, is discussed in Chapter 12, Further Considerations in Planning, and in Chapter 15, Working with Groups. Another area, stages of development, is discussed here in relation to individual therapy.

Stages of Development

Individual therapy goes through stages of development that are similar to the stages discussed for groups in the previous chapter. There are many ways to conceive of stages of development in the therapy relationship. Most of these take into account both natural development through stages and the role of the therapist in helping to achieve what needs to be done at each successive stage.

A four-stage model of the helping process, with tasks to be accomplished in each stage, is provided by Corey and Corey (2015). In the first stage, *identifying clients' problems,* therapists help clients to define and clarify the problems that they would like to address in the context of the therapeutic relationship. In the second stage, *helping clients create goals,* clients are helped to devise new approaches to dealing with their problems. In the third stage, *encouraging clients to take action,* therapists help clients to plan and carry out action strategies for achieving their goals. Finally, in the fourth stage, *termination,* the goal is to help the client to terminate the professional relationship and continue to make the changes on his or her own.

Following is an example of applying this four-stage process. Sam, a medical patient, is referred for assistance in coping with a lengthy hospital stay. The first stage, identifying the problems, begins early in the first session when, as a part of assessment, Sam describes his lengthy disability from a slip on the ice, which caused back problems. This injury led to surgery that has now resulted in a need for painful rehabilitation to enable him to resume his normal activity. The second stage, helping to create goals, is accomplished as Sam identifies his goal as managing the pain of his rehabilitation exercises and coping with being confined in the hospital. In the third stage, encouraging client action, Sam is taught to use music-based relaxation for managing pain. He is also engaged in a songwriting experience in which he writes a verse about what is happening to him, followed by a verse that describes his strengths for coping with the realities of his hospital stay. Sam is encouraged to continue creating lyrics for use in future sessions and given music to support his pain management practices. After several sessions, Sam has developed the ability to create lyrics and melodies to express his feelings about his hospital stay and to use music-based relaxation exercises independently to manage his pain. In the fourth stage, termination, Sam processes the meaning of his hospital and music therapy experience and is encouraged to continue using his new coping skills after discharge.

Bruscia (1987) suggests four main stages in the interpersonal process. In the first stage, *developing a relationship,* the therapist and client find ways to work together. This includes the therapist's work to develop trust and fulfill the client's immediate needs and the client's efforts to find a comfortable way of expressing him- or herself and communicating with the therapist. Conscious thoughts and feelings are explored at a surface level, while unconscious thoughts are explored after a trusting relationship has been established. In the second stage, *conflict resolution,* the relationship that was established in the first stage is used as a means of exploring and working through problems that are at the center of the client's being. During this stage, the client works to bring these problems into awareness. Unconscious material is examined in depth, and new role behaviors are explored but not adopted. In the third stage, *internalization,* the client masters and internalizes the insights and skills that were discovered in the previous stage. Role behaviors are adopted and integrated into the personality. The client is able to make more active, independent choices for his or her life, and the therapist is less active as a helper and serves more as a supportive witness. In the fourth stage, *autonomy,* the client prepares for termination of therapy. Relationships with significant others begin to supplant the need for the therapist. A follow-up plan is agreed upon, and closure is achieved.

Aigen (2005a) describes four experiential states characterized by the interpersonal engagement between client and therapist. *Confusion* can represent the beginning stages of therapy, as the therapist and client are just getting to know each other and how to work together. *Just coping* can refer to challenging moments in therapy that call on the therapist to strive toward resolution without a clear sense of the outcome. *Next best thing* represents a high level of effective and productive work on the part of both client and therapist and can be sustained for extended periods of time. And *real thing* refers to those unpredictable moments, what Maslow would call a peak experience, which are also unsustainable but can propel the work to a new level. These states are not static and do not necessarily move in a linear manner; they can all manifest at various stages in the therapeutic process.

The musical process also unfolds through stages. The client first discovers and learns the sensorimotor schemes of improvising and selects a sound vocabulary for playing and organizing sounds in an intentional way. The sounds being explored become associated with events, feelings, and people in the improviser's experience, leading the improviser to discover how sounds can symbolize both inner experiences and aspects of the external environment. As the improviser develops and repeats short patterns, he or she eventually needs to experience a more complete expression of thoughts and feelings. While musical support from others is initially needed, the improviser later gains control over his or her improvising and the music-making becomes less self-centered. With the increased ability to express him- or herself musically, the improviser begins to desire to share music with others, leading to the need for greater communicativeness. "Music becomes an effective satisfying means of expressing various aspects of the self, meeting psychological and physical needs, and resolving emotional conflicts. Musical interactions with others become a desirable way of learning role behaviors and developing relationships" (Bruscia, 1987, pp. 571–572). Finally, as musical autonomy emerges and the individual gains the ability to maintain his or her musical identity within a group, a personal lifelong relationship with music is established.

Bruscia (1987) describes the stages of improvisational models, applied to both individual and group music therapy. His book, *Improvisational Models of Music Therapy,* can be consulted for help in understanding the developmental process of individual (and group) music therapy. In his summary and synthesis of all of the models, Bruscia suggests that stages of growth in improvisational music therapy can be seen in both the interpersonal and the musical process.

Principles of Facilitating Individual Music Therapy Sessions

Although facilitating individual and group music therapy sessions have many things in common, some principles that apply particularly to individual sessions are described below:

1) Base individual work on a comprehensive assessment that includes medical and diagnostic information; family, job, educational, and social history; psychological history and current state; musical history and preferences; current problems; prognosis; team treatment goals; and anticipated length of treatment.
2) Use music that reflects the client's preferences and musical and social history or cultural background.
3) Have a plan that addresses steps toward established goals but remains open to the possibilities of emerging needs or changes in response patterns.
4) Monitor progress toward goals and collect data as appropriate to the setting.
5) Evaluate progress toward goals and revise at pre-established target dates.
6) Be sensitive to needs which may be identified in music therapy but could more effectively be addressed by another professional and make appropriate referrals.
7) When possible, include the client in treatment planning, evaluation, and goal revision.

Assignments—Working with Individuals

These assignments can help you develop your understanding of working with individuals:

- Consider the clients in your clinical placement. If a client is being seen individually, why was the decision for individual therapy made? How do you think that he or she would progress in a group? If your placement is with a group, choose one client and think about how the music therapy would be different if he or she were receiving individual therapy.
- If you are working with an individual, apply the stages described by Bruscia (1987) of developing a relationship, conflict resolution, internalization, and autonomy, which were discussed earlier in this chapter. Describe the stage in which your client currently is, as well as previous stages through which the therapeutic relationship has progressed. If the stages do not match the stages described by Bruscia, consider why they are different. If you are working with a group, consider how the therapeutic process might be progressing if one of the members were being seen individually.
- If you are working with an individual, consider the four experiential stages of *confusion, just coping, next best thing,* and *real thing* described by Aigen (2005a) and discussed earlier in this chapter. Describe the stage in which your work with your client currently is, as well as previous stages through which the therapeutic relationship has progressed. If you are working with a group, consider how the therapeutic process might be progressing if one of the members were being seen individually. Do this for a specific client.
- Discuss the application of the Principles of Facilitating Individual Music Therapy Sessions for an individual with whom you are working or, if you are not working with an individual, for a person from your group whom you might select for individual treatment. Which of the principles are you following, or would you follow? Discuss their applicability, either in reality or as you think they would be if you were working with this individual.

17 Documentation Strategies

It is important for music therapists to be able to document and communicate what occurs in music therapy. Assessment and evaluation both rely on being able to keep accurate records of how the client is doing. Tallying, duration and latency recording, checklists, rating scales, and interval recording may be used to document client behavior. When using any of these methods, an operational definition—an exact description of the behavior under consideration—will be needed. After we have documented what has taken place, we share this information by writing progress notes. This chapter describes these aspects of documenting and communicating progress.

Documentation is included in the AMTA *Standards of Clinical Practice* and *Professional Competencies*, the CBMT *Board Certification Domains*, and the AMTA/CBMT *Scope of Music Therapy Practice*. It is an integral component of clinical practice; a requirement of employers in meeting legislative, regulatory, and administrative mandates for compliance; and critical for the practitioner in understanding clients and supporting their growth toward health. The article "Clinical Documentation in Music Therapy: Standards, Guidelines, and Laws" (Waldon, 2016) provides a comprehensive discussion and overview of the importance of documentation in relation to our professional standards as well as external bodies.

Operational Definitions

In order to develop measurement systems, the music therapist must first define what is important to measure. Treatment plan goals and objectives delineate what is to be measured. These outcomes must then be defined.

An operational definition outlines a construct (concept) in observable terms. Sheridan and Kratochwill (2010) describe an operational definition as:

> A precise description of the behavior of concern. In general, an effective operational definition meets three important criteria. First, an operational definition should be objective. It should include only observable and measurable characteristics of behavior. Second, it is clear; operational clarity refers to the need for behavior to be defined in terms that are unambiguous, specific, and reliable. A rule of thumb is that the behavior should be explainable to others and should not require interpretation on the part of an observer who was not part of the discussion. Third, an operational discussion must be complete. That is, it should describe what is included and excluded in the behavior, leaving little to the judgment of an independent observer. (p. 33)

It may be helpful to think of an operational definition as a verbal specification of exactly what behaviors will be considered examples of the construct. For example, *agitation* may be operationally defined as "getting out of chair at inappropriate times, pacing around the room, body movements outside of the norm, interrupting the speaker, verbal statements concerning anxiety." Even in this operational definition, there is room for interpretation by the observer. To minimize this, the first step is to make the operational definition as concrete and specific as possible. The second step is to train the observer to bring his or her observations into agreement with what you have in mind a large percentage of the time (i.e., until you have high reliability).

Another type of operational definition is performance on a test or other measure such as a rating scale or behavior checklist. For example, musical ability may be operationally defined as performance on a test of musical ability. Target behaviors may be operationally defined by including specific behaviors on a rating scale or checklist.

Measurement Systems

Once outcomes have been operationally defined, a system for collecting data (measuring response) must be determined. Measurement can include direct and indirect methods. Direct methods involve the music therapist in observing and recording outcome responses. Indirect methods gather information from others involved with the client and may include reports from parents, teachers, or other caregivers.

Direct measures include tests or skills assessment, observational methods, and electronic measures. Krout (2016) describes observational methods used in music therapy, including tallying and frequency recording, duration and latency recording, checklists, rating scales, and interval recording. In tallying, also called frequency or event recording, the observer marks every time that a discrete behavior occurs. This may be done with pencil and paper or a mechanical counter. The important thing is that each incidence of the behavior under consideration is recorded.

In duration recording, the length of time during which something occurs is recorded. This is most accurately done with a stopwatch. Latency recording, which measures the length of time before a behavior occurs, is similar to duration recording.

A checklist is a list of behaviors to be checked off when they occur. Cartwright and Cartwright (1984) suggest that the use of a checklist is appropriate when the behaviors of interest are known in advance and when there is no need to indicate their frequency or quality. Checklists provide information about specific observable behaviors but do not require the therapist to keep count. This is useful when working independently with a group, as it allows the therapist to collect meaningful data over time when counting instances of specific behaviors would not be possible.

A rating scale may be used when the degree or quality of the behavior, trait, or attitude is of interest. One type of rating scale, a Likert scale, is numerical, with numbers corresponding to the degree that the behavior or trait is manifested. Rating scales are by nature less objective than many other forms of measurement because they measure the degree or quality of something, and qualities are not as objective as behaviors.

With interval recording, the time for observation is divided into small intervals (for instance, 15 seconds). Within these intervals, the observer is normally instructed (often via earphones audible only to that person) to observe and to record whether the behavior of interest occurred. Hall and Van Houten (1983) divide interval recording systems into whole or partial interval recording. In whole interval recording, the behavior of interest must occur during the entire interval in order to be counted; in partial interval recording, it is scored if it occurs at all during the interval. Other modes of interval recording include momentary time sampling, a technique to record if a behavior occurs at prespecified time points and *Placheck* recording (i.e., Planned Activity Check), a variation on momentary time sampling (Krout,

2016). Placheck recording, used to collect data about aggregate group behavior, requires the division of the observation period into equal or unequal time periods. At the end of each period, the observer counts the number of group participants engaged in the target behavior in the interval and reports it as a percentage (Ayres & Ledford, 2014). This form of interval recording may be useful in monitoring the response of a group over time.

Madsen and Madsen (1983) suggest that behavior be observed during an initial interval and recorded during the next interval (10-second intervals are recommended). More complex interval recording techniques have been utilized in classroom observations to gather information on teachers and students (Madsen & Madsen; Medley, 1982). These systems utilize codes so that observers can record many different teacher and student behaviors. Interval recording can be used only when a person is available exclusively to observe.

A consideration with any of these measurement systems is the reliability of your measures. You want to have measures that are the same or similar when the data are gathered by several people or at several different points in time (assuming there are no changes in the actual behavior between the two times). A measure of reliability is the correlation between two measures that are taken, and you want the reliability to be high. When the reliability is high, you can trust that the measures would be similar no matter who made them.

Electronic measures include audio- and video-recording. The pioneering work of Paul Nordoff and Clive Robbins included the use of what today might be considered primitive equipment, such as reel-to-reel audio recorders, coupled with still photography and transcribing the recorded music by hand. In addition to transcribing the music, Nordoff and Robbins wrote detailed notes while listening to the recordings of the sessions, a process referred to as "indexing." According to Nordoff and Robbins (2007), indexing recordings can "often reveal events or processes in therapy that were missed or only partially recognized during the actual session. In this way, indexing the recording can serve to broaden, supplement, or even correct impressions gained from the session itself" (p. 182).

For readers who are interested in learning more about various techniques and models of documenting and engaging in detailed analysis of the music in music therapy, we recommend the article "Toward A Practice of Engaged Filming in Nordoff-Robbins Music Therapy" (Graham, 2016) and the book *Microanalysis in Music Therapy: Methods, Techniques and Applications for Clinicians, Researchers, Educators, and Students* (Wosch & Wigram, 2007).

Writing Progress Notes

Following music therapy sessions, it is important to be able to convey what was accomplished. This is generally done in the form of a progress note. Facilities may require progress notes to be written within a specific time frame, or you may get to determine the interval. Many people write progress notes after each session, while at other times, they are done quarterly or at some other selected interval. It is important to record specific observations about the client's responses to interventions in each session so that progress notes written at intervals are based on data and not created from memory, which is quite unreliable.

Progress note requirements have changed with the implementation of the Health Insurance Portability and Accountability Act (HIPAA) in 1996 and the implementation of the Privacy Rule in 2003. The therapist must be careful to document progress toward goals without violating the privacy and confidentiality rights of the client (Wiger, 2012). There are many formats for writing progress notes; some are dictated by a system for planning and documenting sessions that is in effect at the facility. The most commonly used formats for writing notes include SOAP (with sections for subjective, objective, assessment, and plan) and DAP (with sections for data, assessment, and plan) notes. There are variations of these including SOAPIER, DAPE, DARP, and PIRP (Gehart, 2014). These variations are all considered to be problem-oriented approaches to documenting, and thus they can be used to record progress toward goals established in a treatment plan. Learning to write in these formats requires practice and instruction in understanding the intended information for each section. Detailed instruction in the use of SOAP notes can be found in Cameron and Turtle-Song (2002), while Wiger (2012) provides instruction and multiple examples of DAP notes. Both of these are written from a counseling perspective but may be useful to music therapy students learning to write progress notes. Examples of SOAP and DAP notes for music therapy can be found in Tables 17.1 and 17.2.

Table 17.1
Music Therapy Group Note Using SOAP Format

Background information for context for this note (not a part of SOAP):
B is a 45-year-old female living in a long-term care facility after a traumatic brain injury that resulted in physical limitations. She uses a wheelchair for mobility, has limited use of her left side (both upper and lower extremities), and has some word finding difficulty. She received rehabilitative care after her injury but has not progressed to a level of independence that allows her to live outside the facility. She has recently been expressing distress about the possibility of living in an institution indefinitely. This has led to some inappropriate behavior, including arguing with staff, refusing to participate in therapy, and isolation in her room. She was referred to music therapy to address her need to find appropriate avenues of expression for her emotions and to develop coping skills for living in long-term care. As individual music therapy sessions are not available in this facility, she has been attending music therapy group weekly for three weeks at the time of this note.

Sample SOAP note:
9-8-15 1 p.m.
(S) Expressing frustration with living in long-term care and being separated from family and friends. Initially stated "music can't help me feel differently" but by end of session stated she would be back next week. Her lyric contribution, "I get so tired of seeing the same people every day" was sung with enthusiasm.
(O) Resistant to active participation despite coming willingly to group. Responded to preferred music used in session, was singing and helped to write song lyrics. Progressed from minimal response to other group members to asking them for ideas during song writing. Sang new song with enthusiasm.
(A) Despite her frustration and distress, she was able to connect to the music and allow herself to actively participate. Songwriting provided an outlet for her thoughts and feelings about living with a disability.
(P) Continue to include in weekly group with emphasis on self-expression through song writing, improvisation, song choices, and singing.

Table 17.2
Music Therapy Group Note Using DAP Format

Background information for context for this note (not a part of DAP):
M is a mental health consumer, age 37, who has been participating in support programming for two years. She works at a part-time job in the community (with supervision) and attends the support program two days/week. She has been working on developing her ability to notice other persons and focus less on her own concerns.

Sample DAP note:

(D) M arrived early for group. She offered to help prepare the space (distribute song books, move instruments to table) and talked excitedly about being ready to sing. She mentioned she has been thinking of joining the choir at her church but was not sure if she could manage the schedule. In group, she sang with enthusiasm, requested songs, and encouraged others to sing. She chose a hand drum to play during an instrumental improvisation with the group, stating she "liked to help hold the music together with a steady beat." M was animated and smiling through most of the session, with appropriate affective change when another group member was sharing a concern. After the session ended, she stayed to help the therapist put equipment away and confided that when she thinks about joining the church choir, she is worried that she will not be able to sing her part when others are singing something different, as she has not done choral singing since high school.
(A) M was more enthusiastic than usual and more animated. She spoke of her idea to connect to a community group (her church's choir) but expressed uncertainty about the schedule, later revealing her true concern is skill. She was attentive and responsive to other group members and appears to be developing a heightened sense of the needs of others in the group. This is definitely progress from her earlier more self-directed focus in the group.
(P) Monitor M's enthusiasm for singing and her progress in awareness of others. Encourage her to talk about her desire to sing with a group, assisting her in identifying needed resources to make this possible. (MT will include an opportunity to sing a song with different parts, e.g., a round, in next session to begin to build M's skills for moving toward participation in a community music group.)

There is a trend in health care to move all documentation to computerized records, often referred to as Electronic Medical Records (EMR) and Electronic Health Records (EHR). EMRs were developed first and are a computerized version of the standard medical chart in a practice or facility. EHRs include much more than the information from one provider and seek to connect all providers involved in the health-related treatment of an individual. The information travels with the patient and is accessible to the patient, allowing for a more coordinated treatment effort (Garrett & Seidman, 2011). Some therapists still using written notes prefer a template format, as it provides a more efficient way to complete note writing; templates make the shift to computerized records easier. Table 17.3 provides an example of a music therapy progress note using a template style.

Table 17.3
Template-Style Music Therapy Progress Note

Hospice House

Patient _____ (date) _____ (time) _____ Session length _____

Referral source _____ Referral reason _____

Others present _____ LOS @ referral _____

Problems/needs identified _____

Goals addressed:

_____ Increase relaxation _____ Increase interpersonal communication _____ Increase self-expression

_____ Decrease pain _____ Decrease distress/depression _____ Decrease maladaptive behaviors

_____ Increase independent use of resources _____ Increase comfort _____ Increase spriritual connection

_____ Increase contact with here and now _____ Mobilize coping skills

_____ End of life support _____ (other) _____

Interventions used:

___ Song choice ___ Singing to ___ Singing with ___ Patient solo ___ Group singing

___ Receptive listening ___ To recorded music ___ To live music ___ Music-assisted relaxtion

___ Lyric or music evoked reminiscing ___ Reality orientation ___ Rhythmic engagement

___ Songwriting ___ Compsoing ___ Improvisation ___ Vocal ___ Instrumental

Other _____

Narrative report:

Therapist signature & title _____

It is common in many settings to use abbreviations in note writing. Many facilities have a list of approved abbreviations to be used in notes. However, research suggests that this common practice of abbreviating, especially when care is being provided by a multidisciplinary team, is counterproductive and easily misunderstood and could lead to errors in treatment (Parvaiz, Subramanian, & Kendall, 2008; Sinha, McDermott, Srinivas, & Houghton, 2011). Music therapy students are cautioned to use only abbreviations that are approved for use in your particular setting and to write out anything that could be misinterpreted.

Table 17.4 contains a sample of what needs to be included in a narrative progress note.

Table 17.4
Music Therapy Progress Note
(Data-Based Narrative Note)

Client Information
Name (may be coded in some learning situations to protect confidentiality)
Facility
Age or date of birth
Diagnoses (list in order of importance; if they are numerous, may select the most pertinent)
Number of sessions attended out of number available
Initial behavior (describe how client behaved when sessions began)

Overview of Music Therapy
Goals
Objectives
Sample procedures (intended to make it clear to anyone who reads the note how the sample
procedures are designed to work on the goals and objectives)
Progress (toward each goal)

Signature and Title

Table 17.5 provides an example of this progress note format as it might be written for an actual client. In reviewing progress toward goals, you want to include information that describes the quality of the client's level of participation in the music therapy experiences, as well as any interventions used to motivate that participation, such as encouraging, cuing, or assisting.

Be sure to describe what the client did in the session, such as singing; verbalizing about memories, feelings, or ideas; playing instruments; imitating rhythms; creating melody or rhythms; improvising; interacting with others; or contributing to group projects such as songwriting.

A progress note also includes how the client responded to the therapist. Be sure to note if the client made eye contact, was verbal or nonverbal, initiated interaction, sought attention, offered assistance, and was cooperative or enthusiastic about the experience. Additionally, you will want to make note of any other factors that influenced the client's participation and responses, or anything that distinguishes the client's participation. If you are dealing with a client who exhibits inappropriate behaviors in the session, make note of what you did in response to these behaviors and what was successful or not successful. If the client was agitated, distressed, or withdrawn, what do you know about the source of this response and what were you able to do to draw him or her into the music therapy experience?

Progress notes may be of varying lengths, depending upon the requirements of your setting and the needs of your clients. The most important function of a progress note is to document what the client did, how the therapist intervened, and how the client responded to intervention. A progress note should be clear and concise but include enough detail that another staff member can get a picture of how the client is progressing in music therapy and what has worked or not worked thus far.

Table 17.5
Sample Narrative Music Therapy Progress Note

Client Information

Name: Linda
Facility: Nursing Home in Mytown
Date of birth: DOB: 12/01/34
Diagnoses: Dementia, cause unknown; depression (dysthemia)
Number of sessions attended out of number available: 10 out of 12
Initial behavior: When the sessions began, Linda tended to be lethargic. She did not interact with the therapist or any of the other residents. She seldom initiated any kind of response and had to be cajoled to participate. She seemed quite confused and did not know the day of the week or where she was. She was willing to remain in the session but did little else. She was observed reaching up to rearrange her hair, demonstrating that she could lift her arms.

Overview of Music Therapy

Goal: Increase verbal interaction
Sample objective: During planned break in lyrics of song, client will face another client and answer the question posed by the song with a maximum of one prompt.
Goal: Improve range of motion
Sample objective: During music and movement activity, client will move arms in direction up or down as modeled by therapist, with at least 12-inch movement between the two directions.
Sample procedures: All music therapy sessions followed a similar format and included an opening experience intended to encourage verbal interaction. The main part of the session consisted of one or more musical strategies such as singing, playing simple instruments, and/or composing a song, and always included some movement. All procedures built upon the social aspects of music. Sessions concluded with a brief recapitulation of what had been done in the session and a closing song.
Progress: Linda made progress toward the first goal, increase verbal interaction. In 8 of the 10 sessions that she attended, she faced another client and answered the question posed by the song with a maximum of one prompt. On two occasions, she spontaneously spoke with the music therapist. She made substantial progress toward the second goal, improve range of motion, being able to accurately imitate the therapists' movement on 7 out of 10 sessions within the targeted range.

Lucy Smith, Music Therapy Student
Signature and Title

Assignments—Documentation Strategies

These assignments should help you to develop your documentation skills:

- Devise two observation methods using the measurement systems described in this chapter. If you are observing, create a hypothetical clinical setting and describe how you would use the tools. If you are working in a practicum setting where you are able to collect data, use these measurement systems in the session. If you are able to record the data yourself, you should do so. If you need assistance from someone else, find a way to get that assistance. Report the results in a way that is comprehensible to someone who did not attend the session.
- Look at the goals that you have selected for your session. Are there words or phrases for which the meanings are not completely clear (perhaps *reality orientation* or *range of motion*)? Even if you think that the words are clear, reviewing will be useful practice in writing operational definitions. Choose three words or phrases from a recent session plan. Ask several people to read the operational definitions and see if they have the same idea that you do. An operational definition is acceptable only when the words are clear and understood the same by everyone involved.
- Write a progress note for one of the clients in your clinical setting using the SOAP format.
- Write a progress note using the DAP format.

18 Self-Assessment for the Music Therapist

This chapter focuses on the music therapist rather than on the client. It will offer some ideas about the importance of continuous growth, some directions for growth, and some tools to continue your growth throughout your career. "It is possible for you to become an effective, intentional therapist. Helping can be a way of life, but it requires the ability to change, grow, and develop with your clients" (Ivey & Simek-Downing, 1980, p. 14). How *does* a therapist change, grow, and develop with his or her clients? The first step is self-assessment. We begin the process of self-assessment as music therapy students and will continue it throughout our professional lives. This self-assessment helps each music therapist to develop "the effective use of the self in the 'now' ... generated by what has been learned and recognized within the self" (Baldwin, 2013, p. 10). Baldwin goes on to elaborate on the benefits of making changes in our personal life as a way of freeing energy to work with clients and deepening our ability to empathize with client distress. This ability to reflect on how we move through life, what experiences and factors have influenced our way of being, and our understanding of those influences is defined as "reflexivity." Reflexivity is central to helping the client grow and requires that the therapist "make continuous efforts to bring into awareness, evaluate, and, when necessary, modify his work with a client before, during, and after each session, as well as at various stages of the therapy process ... through self-observation, self-inquiry, collaboration with the client, consultation with experts, and professional supervision" (Bruscia, 2014b, p. 36).

Various authors have written about this process. Hanser (2016) has addressed the journey to becoming a music therapist from a holistic perspective in *Integrative Health Through Music Therapy*. Resources from outside of music therapy include *The Making of a Therapist: A Practical Guide to the Inner Journey* by Cozolino (2004); *How Can I Help? Stories and Reflections on Service* by Dass and Gorman (1985); *How Therapists Change: Personal and Professional Reflections* by Goldfried (2001); *On Becoming a Psychotherapist: The Personal and Professional Journey* by Klein, Bernard, and Schermer (2011); *Therapeutic Mastery: Becoming a More Creative and Effective Therapist* by Kramer (2000); *Effective Helping: Interviewing and Counseling Techniques,* 8th edition, by Okun and Kantrowitz (2015); and *Becoming an Effective Therapist* by Sperry, Carlson, and Kjor (2003). An article that addresses arts therapies is "Therapist Self-Awareness: An Essential Tool in Music Therapy" by Camilleri (2001).

The Process of Self-Assessment

During coursework and clinical training, the AMTA *Professional Competencies* (2013a) are a guide to developing skills required to become a qualified music therapist. These competencies define needed development in the areas of music foundations, clinical foundations, and music therapy. The competencies can be used not only to track student progress in academic work but also as a means of self-assessment, assisting the student in identifying areas that need attention during training. Following training, it is reasonable to assert that not every competency will be mastered at the same level, so this document may still be useful in identifying areas for continued growth. Further guidance, as one gains experience and/or additional education, may be found in the AMTA *Advanced Competencies* (American Music Therapy Association, 2015a), which define skills and knowledge related to professional practice and professional development at a more advanced level. These documents present an expectation that a competent music therapist will have developed music skills and therapy skills that allow the therapist to meet the needs of clients at a supportive level for entry-level therapists and at a more complex level for those meeting advanced competencies. A plan for self-growth can be developed using these documents.

Music therapists also need to develop verbal therapy skills in addition to their music skills. As you continue to grow as a therapist, you will want to monitor your own development in this area. In order to do so, you will need to self-assess specific skills. Okun and Kantrowitz (2015) emphasize the importance of listening, attending, perceiving, and responding as components of communication that allow therapy to progress. Sperry, Carlson, and Kjor (2003) define factors needed in therapy to include (a) empathy; (b) engagement of the client, which is broken into component parts such as attending, active listening, empathic response, and encouragement; (c) negotiating goals and treatment; (d) seeding hope; and (e) triggering the placebo effect, which is a reflection of the client's faith in the therapist and/or treatment process (p. 34).

The importance of developing verbal skills might best be understood from Pennebaker's (1997) view of music therapy:

> Dance, art, and music therapies can be powerful in getting individuals to experience emotions related to relevant upheavals in their lives .... Indeed, most dance, art, and music therapists go far beyond encouraging self-expression. During or after dancing, drawing, or singing, clients are strongly encouraged to talk about their emotional experiences. In other words, non–language-based therapies rely heavily on language once the clients' inhibitions are lifted. (p. 101)

How can you as a music therapist in training (and later as a music therapist in practice) learn about yourself? What tools and resources do you have to help you to assess the skills and knowledge necessary for effective clinical work? While you are a student, you have instructors and clinical supervisors to offer you feedback. Once you are a practicing therapist, you can seek supervision or a mentor to help you examine your work, support you as you develop a better understanding of your work, and help you settle into the beginnings of your therapeutic style. The value of a supervisor or mentor cannot be stated too strongly. This person can cheer you on when discouraged, hold you up when tired, smile with you in the joy of your successes, and hold you accountable for your needed changes and growth. This valued professional can mean the difference between staying in the field and working with a healthy attitude or leaving music therapy because of burnout.

In addition to external help, you can take responsibility for your own growth by developing the habit of looking at yourself and your work in a systematic manner. The AMTA website houses a self-assessment document based on the *Standards of Practice* designed to assist the music therapist in evaluating the quality of services offered and identifying areas for growth (Stephenson, Long, Oswanski, Plancon, Pujol, Smith-Morse, & Gainsfera, 2008).

Bruscia (2001) offers a five-level model for supervision that might be adapted to your self-assessment as follows:

1) *Action-oriented:* Do you need to do something differently?
2) *Learning-oriented:* Do you need to acquire knowledge, skill, or insight in order to

address a problem or weakness in your work?

3) *Client-oriented:* Do you need to understand your client differently?

4) *Experience-oriented:* Can you reframe the way you experience the therapy process with the client?

5) *Countertransference-oriented:* Are there personal issues involved in your work with this client or group?

As a self-reflective music therapy student, you can ask yourself these questions and seek assistance from teachers and supervisors as needed. This will help you to develop the habit of examining yourself and your work, a habit that will serve you well in your development and growth as a therapist throughout your career.

Thinking About Self-Assessment

In order to make self-assessment meaningful, you may want to begin to think about it as soon as you start to assist with sessions. Keeping a log or journal that catalogs and gives a chronology of your experiences and also includes your reactions, responses, questions, and concerns is the foundation for self-assessment. You may find that you naturally begin to identify specific skills that you need to develop. You can take responsibility for making a plan to develop those skills, including seeking out classes, lessons, practice sessions, or readings that will help you to address these needs. In the following example, a music therapy student is assisting with groups in her clinical practicum. She identifies a weakness in her skills and plans to address it:

> I'm assisting with sessions at a daycare center for frail older adults with both physical and cognitive dysfunction. My piano skills are good enough to accompany group singing, and I'm really excited that I've been asked by the supervising therapist, Jane, to plan to accompany the sing-along portion of the session. Jane provided me with a list of four songs to be used in the next session and told me that I should be sure the music I use to accompany the songs does not have any melody notes that are higher than C. I've searched for music at school and found that one of the songs is too high and has to be transposed. I didn't really have enough time in my schedule to write out the transposition, so I penciled in the melody notes and wrote the chords above, hoping I would be able to play it for my clinical assignment. When I played the song for the group to sing, I kind of stumbled along and the group didn't sing as much on this song as on the others. They weren't as animated, and I had to work really hard just to get through the song. I've decided to set aside an hour each week to practice playing songs in different keys, beginning by transposing down a third, fourth, or fifth in order to improve my skills.

Consider how you think about yourself as a therapist. What role do you see yourself playing in your therapeutic relationship with clients? Do you see yourself as a facilitator, helper, and guide, or are you caught up in a need to save people who need your help? Do you see yourself as the person with the knowledge or *right* answers? Do you know what is best for the clients and make all the decisions? Recognizing the differing advantages of both directive and nondirective approaches can provide a more balanced and effective process. Be sensitive to the timing of what occurs in sessions, to the flow of the music, and to the pace of growth. Ivey and Simek-Downing (1980) suggest that, if we can understand the world from the client's point of view, we are more likely to make effective choices in our therapeutic interactions. Maslow (1999) proposes getting into the *Weltanschauung* (a German term meaning "worldview") of the client—in essence, seeing the world through the eyes of your client.

How do you see your actions? How do you decide what to do when? This book is filled with information about how to think about, plan for, and implement music therapy sessions. Reflect on how your work compares to the suggestions made in this book. Take time to review your own work and attitudes toward your work and allow yourself to grow. Be conscious of doing so on a regular basis, not engaging in this kind of self-reflection only when it is assigned by your instructor or clinical supervisor. Be curious and exploratory in what you want to know about yourself as a musician and as a therapist.

How do you think about your clients? How do you understand them and the behaviors they exhibit? Be sensitive to the typical characteristics of each illness or disability. Be knowledgeable about the steps of normal development and develop your observation skills and clinical intuitions so that you recognize developmentally appropriate changes as they occur. Be alert to recognizing when your perceptions of the client or the therapy process are affected by your own life experiences and understanding. Take time to become familiar with who you are and what experiences have influenced and formed you.

Hanser (2016) invites readers to adopt a holistic view of the therapy process that requires self-exploration. As she describes the therapist's joining with the client (to whom she refers as the "person"), she suggests that one must first know one's self. She presents a series of preparation exercises for increasing self-knowledge that enable you to bring your whole self into the clinical session as you walk with that client in the journey from illness to wellness.

Tools for Self-Assessment

Journaling

This conscious effort to write about your experiences can be most helpful. Pennebaker (1997) suggests that to write about content in the context of your own feelings, thoughts, hopes, and other subjective experiences in relation to what happens during sessions is more powerful than talking or writing about the content alone. Thus, journaling about clinical experiences can be an effective way to learn about the clinical therapy process and to grow as a therapist and as a person. In order for journaling to be effective, the journal needs to address some specific topics. Your instructor may choose a specific model for journaling that is used for class assignments, but you may find another format more effective for your own use.

Journals may include (a) an objective chronology of the experience; (b) a subjective summary of your responses to the experience; (c) an observational focus on client response; (d) a focus on a particular theme or topic, for instance, use of music skills in a particular session or what my client might have been thinking as the session progressed; (e) an evaluation of the effectiveness of the session; (f) a post session review of the plan as compared to the actual session process; (g) ideas for future interventions; and (h) comparison to a specific model or theory of music therapy.

Journals are also more useful if we return to them after a period of time and, as we reread them, look for growth and learning. You may find it useful to read a semester's worth of entries and summarize your own learning. You might also include unresolved issues, questions, and skills that you have not yet developed. This unfinished business may become a part of your journaling process in the next semester. Taking the time to write reflexively about your experiences and perceptions followed by a review of these thoughts can lead to a deeper understanding of underlying assumptions and beliefs as well as solidify connections between theoretical knowledge and practical application.

Journaling is not something that should stop when classes are over. Continue journaling during your breaks, during the summer, and, perhaps even more important, during your internship and on into your life as a professional music therapist. It can be an invaluable tool to aid you in continuing your own self-assessment and reflection.

Work Sheets

Some people find it useful to have a form to fill out to help them think about their work. You may find the format suggested below for self-reflective exercises to be easier to use than journaling and reflecting on the questions found above. Use those that are most helpful to you at this time in your growth, recognizing that some questions may be more relevant later on or that some may not apply to you.

Many students will want to transfer these work sheets to their computer and to answer the questions using the computer. You are encouraged to do this if it will help you to take full advantage of the work sheets. Two examples of the work sheet format for self-reflective exercises follow. *Note:* These exercises may stir feelings or require further elaboration by someone with more knowledge and/or experience or may need to be brought to a supervision session. Don't try to resolve issues raised by self-reflection alone; discuss your thoughts and feelings with your site supervisor, faculty supervisor, or personal therapist. Music therapists have an ethical responsibility to engage in whatever self-care will permit them to keep their own emotional life in balance in order to be available to the client. Seek help when you need it.

"That Client"

Some clients stir emotional responses in us as we work with them. This may be a result of our lack of understanding about the nature of the illness or disability, it may be that we have expectations that are mismatched to the capacities of the client, or it may be that this client stirs some personal issues in us (countertransference). We can learn from this experience by taking the time to examine our own responses.

1) When in the session did I notice myself reacting or responding to the client in a manner that was inconsistent with good therapy? What was the client doing? What was happening musically? What was I doing?
2) Do I understand what behaviors or responses are within normal limits for this particular client? How does his or her diagnosis or challenge affect the responses I see in music therapy? What is developmentally appropriate for this client?
3) What goals were set for this client? Did I set them alone or with input from other professionals, or did the client have a role in setting them? Did I get enough information at assessment to be clear about what this client needs and what he or she is capable of doing?
4) Does this client want to be in music therapy? Is this client motivated to change? Did the client make the decision to seek treatment or was the decision made by a parent or guardian, and how does that affect the client's motivation to participate in the therapy experience?
5) Are there qualities about this client or my perception of this client that remind me

of someone from my own life? What is my relationship with that person? Do I have any unresolved issues in that relationship? Am I projecting aspects of that relationship onto this client?

Post Session Review

It is always useful to spend some time to review a music therapy session. The steps outlined here may help in this process but are just one way to do a review. You may find other ways that are more effective for you.

1) Describe the flow of your session. What form or structure did you use? Was there a beginning, middle, and end to the session? How did you open the session? How did you introduce the focus of the session? How did you close? Did it serve as closure to the experience?
2) Describe your work as the facilitator/leader. How directive were you in the group process? When directions for an experience were required? Were you clear about what the clients were to do? Did you use as few words as possible so that the clients could process without extra words? How clear was your role to clients? How clear were the clients' roles to themselves? How well did you incorporate the factors that encourage therapy to progress—empathy, engagement, including the clients in goal-planning, and seeding hope that change is possible?
3) How did the clients respond to the session? Were they easily engaged in the music experiences? Did they interact freely with the therapist? Did they interact with one another in a group setting? When applicable, were clients able to articulate some benefit that they received from participating?
4) Where do you go from here? What does this client or group need to do next to work toward the established goals? Are there materials that you need to incorporate? Are there skills that you need to acquire?
5) Write about your session. What stands out in your mind? What is it about that particular experience that draws your attention? Can you write about the emotional, cognitive, or physical responses you have to the experience? What might this be related to in your life?

Personal Therapy

Undergoing your own personal therapy is one of the best ways to continue growing. Many campuses provide access to psychotherapy, so this may be something that you can pursue while you are still studying. Some music therapy students and music therapists begin their own therapy because they feel that this is a good way to learn what therapy is about. This is certainly true. However, most people who begin therapy with this in mind find that as they go through the process, they also have legitimate problems and issues that they are able to deal with in therapy.

Of course, there are many different models of therapy. Keep these in mind when choosing a therapist and follow a model of therapy that is congruent with your personal beliefs and one that will meet your needs.

Music therapy students and music therapists often decide to engage in music therapy as clients. This may be psychotherapeutically oriented music therapy. Music therapy may also be accessed in addition to traditional psychotherapy. Some music therapy training programs include an experiential music therapy component (see Murphy & Wheeler, 2005), and students in these programs may have had a music therapy experience that was therapeutic in addition to being educational. This should not be considered a substitute for either music therapy or psychotherapy but may provide a good opportunity for growth as well as a model for music therapy.

Using Music for Self-Assessment

Since music is the primary tool in our therapy work, it is appropriate and desirable to use music as a tool for self-growth. Music might be used improvisationally, re-creatively, compositionally, or receptively. Just as with the work sheet suggestions above, these exercises may stir feelings or require further elaboration by someone with more knowledge and/or experience or may need to be brought to a supervision session. Don't try to resolve issues raised by self-reflection alone; discuss your thoughts and feelings with your site supervisor, faculty supervisor, or personal therapist.

The tools offered here are for self-reflection and the professional growth of the therapist and not intended for use in your clinical work. Before using these self-reflective musical experiences with clients, be sure that you have had adequate training and experience and have access to supervision.

Improvisational Tools

1) Think about a client relationship that you wish to understand more deeply. Choose an instrument that will allow you to metaphorically describe the client through sound. You might want to tape yourself in order to more effectively listen to what you create when you are expressing the client through your own music. Listen reflectively, allowing yourself to hear the music from different perspectives. Describe the music, your response to it, the qualities that it has. How do these relate to your understanding of the client? How do these relate to your understanding of yourself?

2) You might also create a dialogue between the client and yourself by choosing two instruments, one to represent the client and one to represent yourself, and then playing. Reflective listening to a tape recording of this music may help you to gain insight into the relationship. Describe the qualities of the music, your responses to it, and the interaction between the sounds. What does this reveal about the relationship, the client, and you?

Re-creative Tools

1) Choose a song or piece that you love to perform, then perform it with enthusiasm. When you finish, journal about the experience of performing. Reconnect with why you love music, and write about why you believe in the power of music to change others. How does this reflection affect your view of your clinical work?

2) Join a community performance group and participate with a dual intention. While participating in the rehearsals and performances, be aware of how you are responding to the music, to the group, to the conductor, to the audience. What can you learn about yourself and your relationship to music? How does this affect your skills in the clinical environment?

Compositional Tools

1) Write a song about your client, group, or session experience or a particular issue with which you are struggling in your growth. You might use lyrics or not; you might write for only one instrument or perhaps more than one. If you are reflecting on a group experience, lyrics or multiple instruments might be more effective than a single line melody. Tap into your musical self to gain a deeper understanding of your therapist self.

2) Write a poem about your therapy work and then orchestrate it with sounds or music. Perform it for yourself. Consider taping it and doing some reflective listening when you are done.

Receptive Tools

1) Take time away from your academic and clinical work to listen to music that you especially enjoy. Allow yourself to be as completely involved in the music as you can, using the musical experience as a respite from the hard work of learning and becoming. Return to your work and notice how you are now approaching it. Has your perspective changed? Do you notice changes in your energy level? Do you have the motivation to continue your work?

2) Practice relaxation exercises with music. If you have not yet learned to do this, find a taped version and use it. (Your instructor may make a recommendation.) In this relaxed state, revisit your clinical experience to see if your perceptions have changed.

3) Choose a recording that reflects how you are feeling and listen to it. Allow yourself to experience the emotion in the music. After listening, take time to write about the experience, identifying any insights that you may gain.

Assignments—Self-Assessment

Along with the strategies and tools for self-assessment already outlined above, the following assignments will assist you in further deepening your understanding of self-assessment:

- Select one of the tools under Using Music for Self-Assessment, then carry out one of the exercises under that tool. Write about your experience and discuss with your supervisor.
- Use the AMTA *Professional Competencies* to assess your current level of competence.
- Select a work sheet question that is relevant to your current placement. Write out the answers and discuss your responses with someone else involved in music therapy—a classmate, supervisor, or teacher.
- If you used journal writing during your placement, review your entries near the end of the semester to identify any changes in perspective, understanding, or awareness that you have developed.
- Self-assessment is an ongoing process. It is essential to all therapists' growth and development. We continue to grow and develop throughout our careers. As you near the completion of your training to be a music therapist, begin to make self-assessment part of your own process.
- Discover the tools that are most useful for you. Use several of them as you lead your music therapy sessions. Continue to revisit this chapter after your formal academic work is completed and you are a practicing music therapist.

References

Abbott, E. (2015). Characterizing objective observations in music therapy: A study of student practicum logs. *Music Therapy Perspectives.* Advance online publication. doi:10.1093/mtp/miv037

Adler, R. (2001). *Musical Assessment of Gerontologic Needs and Treatment: The MAGNET Survey.* St. Louis, MO: MMB Music.

Ahonen-Eerikäinen, H. (2007). *Group Analytic Music Therapy.* Gilsum, NH: Barcelona.

Aigen, K. (1991). The roots of music therapy: Towards an indigenous research paradigm. (Doctoral dissertation, New York University, 1990). *Dissertation Abstracts International, 52*(6), 1933A.

Aigen, K. (1995). An aesthetic foundation of clinical theory: An underlying basis of creative music therapy. In C. Kenny (Ed.), *Listening, playing, creating: Essays on the power of sound* (pp. 233–257). Albany, NY: State University of NY Press.

Aigen, K. (1997). *Here we are in music: One year with an adolescent Creative Music Therapy group.* St. Louis, MO: MMB Music.

Aigen, K. (1998). *Paths of development in Nordoff-Robbins Music Therapy.* Gilsum, NH: Barcelona.

Aigen, K. (2002). *Playin' in the band: A qualitative study of popular music styles as clinical improvisation.* New York, NY: Nordoff-Robbins Center for Music Therapy, New York University.

Aigen, K. (2005a). *Being in music: Foundations of Nordoff-Robbins Music Therapy.* Gilsum, NH: Barcelona.

Aigen, K. (2005b). *Music-Centered Music Therapy.* Gilsum, NH: Barcelona.

Aigen, K. (2014a). Music-centered dimensions of Nordoff-Robbins music therapy. *Music Therapy Perspectives, 32*(1), 18–29. doi:10.1093/mtp/miu006

Aigen, K. (2014b). *The study of music therapy: Current issues and concepts.* New York, NY: Rutledge.

Ainsworth, M. S., & Bowlby, J. (1991). An ethological approach to personality development. *American Psychologist, 46*(4), 333–341. doi:10.1037/0003-066X.46.4.333

Aldridge, D. (1996). *Music therapy research and practice in medicine: From out of the silence.* Philadelphia, PA: Jessica Kingsley.

Aldridge, G. (1996). "A walk through Paris": The development of melodic expression in music therapy with a breast-cancer patient. *Arts in Psychotherapy, 23*(3), 207–223. doi:10.1016/0197-4556(96)00024-Xdoi:10.1016/0197-4556(96)00024-X

American Music Therapy Association. (2013a). *Professional Competencies.* Retrieved from www.musictherapy.org/about/competencies/

American Music Therapy Association. (2013b). *Standards of Clinical Practice.* Retrieved from www.musictherapy.org/about/standards/

American Music Therapy Association. (2014a). *Code of Ethics.* Retrieved from www.musictherapy.org/about/ethics/

American Music Therapy Association. (2014b). *Standards for Education and Clinical Training.* Retrieved from www.musictherapy.org/members/edctstan/

American Music Therapy Association. (2015a). *Advanced Competencies.* Retrieved from www.musictherapy.org/members/advancedcomp/

American Music Therapy Association. (2015b). Certification Board for Music Therapists. *Scope of Music Therapy Practice.* Retrieved from www.musictherapy.org/about/scope_of_music_therapy_practice/; www.cbmt.org/ (home; Scope of Music Therapy Practice)

American Psychiatric Association. (2013). *Diagnostic and statistical manual of mental disorders* (5ᵗʰ ed.). Arlington, VA: American Psychiatric Publishing.

Amir, D. (1996). Music therapy—Holistic model. *Music Therapy, 14*(1), 44–60. doi:10.1093/mt/14.1.44

Amir, D. (2001a). How do we nurture ourselves? *Voices Resources.* Retrieved from http://testvoices.uib.no/community/?q=fortnightly-columns/2001-how-do-we-nurture-ourselves

Amir, D. (2001b). Sometimes, it is our task to find out how much music we can still make with what we have left. *Voices Resources.* Retrieved from https://voices.no/community/?q=fortnightly-columns/2001-sometimes-it-our-task-find-out-how-much-music-we-can-still-make-what-we-hav

Ansdell, G. (2001). Musicology: Misunderstood guest at the music therapy table? In G. D. Franco, E. Ruud, T. Wigram, & D. Aldridge (Eds.), *Music Therapy in Europe* (pp. 17–34). The Fifth European Music Therapy Conference, Naples, Italy. Rome, Italy: ISMEZ.

Asmus, E. P. (1985). The development of a multidimensional instrument for the measurement of affective responses to music. *Psychology of Music, 13*(1), 19–30. doi:10.1177/0305735685131002

Austin, D. (1999). Vocal improvisation in analytically oriented music therapy with adults. In T. Wigram & J. De Backer (Eds.), *Clinical applications of music therapy in psychiatry* (pp. 141–157). Philadelphia, PA: Jessica Kingsley.

Austin, D. (2008). *The theory and practice of vocal psychotherapy: Songs of the self.* London, UK: Jessica Kingsley.

Ayres, K., & Ledford, J. R. (2014). Dependent measures and measurement systems. In D. L. Gast & J. R. Ledford (Eds.), *Single case research methodology: Application in special education and behavioral sciences* (pp. 124-153). New York, NY: Routledge.

Baker, F. (2005). Working with impairments in pragmatics through songwriting with traumatically brain-injured patients. In F. Baker & T. Wigram (Eds.), *Songwriting: Methods, techniques and clinical applications for music therapy clinicians, educators, and students* (pp. 134–153). London, UK: Jessica Kingsley.

Baker, F., & Wigram, T. (Eds.). (2005). *Songwriting. Methods, techniques and clinical applications for music therapy clinicians, educators, and students.* London, UK: Jessica Kingsley.

Baker, F. A. (2015). *Therapeutic songwriting: Developments in theory, methods, and practice.* London, UK: Palgrave Macmillan.

Baker, F. A., & Ballantyne, J. (2013). "You've got to accentuate the positive": Group songwriting to promote a life of enjoyment, engagement and meaning in again Australians. *Nordic Journal of Music Therapy, 22*(1), 7–24. doi:10.1080/08098131.2012.678372

Baker, F. A., Silverman, M. J., & MacDonald, R. (2016). Reliability and validity of the meaningfulness of songwriting scale (MSS) with adults on acute psychiatric and detoxification units. *Journal of Music Therapy, 53*(1), 55–74. doi:10.1093/jmt/thv020

Baldwin, M. (2013). *The use of self in therapy* (3ʳᵈ ed.). New York, NY: Routledge.

Ball, T. S., & Bernadoni, L. C. (1953). The application of an auditory apperception test to clinical diagnosis. *Journal of Clinical Psychology, 9*(1), 54–58. doi:10.1002/1097-4679(195301)9:1<54::AID-JCLP2270090116>3.0.CO;2-X

Bandura, A. (1963). *Social learning and personality development*. New York, NY: Holt, Rinehart, and Winston.

Baxter, H. T., Berghofer, J. A., MacEwan, L., Nelson, J., Peters, K., & Roberts, P. (2007). *The Individualized Music Therapy Assessment Profile, IMTAP*. London, UK: Jessica Kingsley.

Benjamin, A. (2001). *The helping interview, with case illustrations*. Boston, MA: Houghton Mifflin.

Berger, D. S. (2009). On developing music therapy goals and objectives. *Voices: A World Forum for Music Therapy, 9*(1). Retrieved from https://voices.no/index.php/voices/article/view/362/285. doi:10.15845/voices.v9i1.362

Berman, I. (1981). Musical functioning, speech lateralization, and the amusias. *South African Medical Journal, 59*, 78–81.

Bitcon, C. H. (2000). *Alike and different* (2nd ed.). Gilsum, NH: Barcelona.

Blacking, J. (1973). *How musical is man?* Seattle, WA: University of Washington Press.

Bogue, R. (2005). Use S.M.A.R.T. goals to launch management by objectives plan. *TechRepublic*. Retrieved from www.techrepublic.com/article/use-smart-goals-to-launch-management-by-objectives-plan/

Bolton, R. (1979). *People skills*. New York, NY: Simon & Schuster.

Bonde, L. (2011). Health musicing: Music therapy or music and health? *Music and Arts in Action, 3*(2), 120–140.

Bonny, H. (1980). *GIM therapy: Past, present and future implications*. Salina, KS: The Bonny Foundation.

Bonny, H. (2002). *Music and consciousness: The evolution of Guided Imagery and Music*. Gilsum, NH: Barcelona.

Borczon, R. M. (1997). *Music therapy: Group vignettes*. Gilsum, NH: Barcelona.

Borling, J. (2011). Music therapy and addiction: Addressing essential components in the recovery process. In A. Meadows (Ed.), *Developments in music therapy practice: Case study examples* (pp. 334–349). Gilsum, NH: Barcelona.

Boxill, E. H. (1985). *Music therapy for the developmentally disabled*. Rockville, MD: Aspen Systems Corporation.

Boxill, E. H. (1997). *The miracle of music therapy*. Gilsum, NH: Barcelona.

Boyle, M. E., & Krout, R. (1987). *Music therapy clinical training manual*. St. Louis, MO: MMB Music.

Brammer, L. M., & MacDonald, G. (2003). *The helping relationship: Process and skills* (8th ed.). Boston, MA: Allyn & Bacon.

Braswell, C., Brooks, D. M., DeCuir, A., Humphrey, T., Jacobs, K. W., & Sutton, K. (1983). Development and implementation of a music/activity therapy intake assessment for psychiatric patients. Part I: Initial standardization procedures on data from university students. *Journal of Music Therapy, 20*(2), 88–100. doi:10.1093/jmt/20.2.88

Braswell, C., Brooks, D. M., DeCuir, A., Humphrey, T., Jacobs, K. W., & Sutton, K. (1986). Development and implementation of a music/activity therapy intake assessment for psychiatric patients. Part II: Standardization procedures on data from psychiatric patients. *Journal of Music Therapy, 23*(3), 126–141. doi:10.1093/jmt/23.3.126

Braverman, S., & Chevigny, H. (1964). *The Braverman Chevigny Auditory Projective Test*. New York, NY: American Foundation for the Blind.

Briggs, C. (1991). A model for understanding musical development. *Music Therapy, 10*(1), 1–21. doi:10.1093/mt/10.1.1

Briggs, C. A. (2015). Developmental approaches. In B. L. Wheeler (Ed.), *Music therapy handbook* (pp. 172–182). New York, NY: Guilford Press.

Briggs, C. A., & Bruscia, K. (1985, November). *Developmental models for understanding music behavior.* Paper presented at the Joint Conference on the Creative Arts Therapists, National Coalition of Arts Therapy Associations, New York, NY.

Bright, R. (1991). *Music in geriatric care: A second look.* Wahroonga, NSW, Australia: Music Therapy Enterprises.

Brotons, M., & Marti, P. (2003). Music therapy with Alzheimer's patients and their family caregivers: A pilot project. *Journal of Music Therapy, 40*(2), 138–150. doi:10.1093/jmt/40.2.138

Broucek, M. (1987). *An interpersonal model of music therapy improvisation.* Unpublished master's thesis, Hahnemann University, Philadelphia, PA.

Brunk, B. (1997). *Songwriting for music therapists.* Grapevine, TX: Prelude Music Therapy.

Brunk, B., & Coleman, K. (2000). Development of a special education music therapy assessment process. *Music Therapy Perspectives, 18*(1), 59–68. doi:10.1093/mtp/18.1.59

Bruscia, K. (1984, April). *Are we losing our identity as music therapists?* Paper presented at the Mid-Atlantic Regional Conference, Philadelphia, PA.

Bruscia, K. (1988). Standards for clinical assessment in the arts therapies. *Arts in Psychotherapy, 15*(1), 5–10. doi:10.1016/0197-4556(88)90047-0

Bruscia, K. (2000). A scale for assessing responsiveness to Guided Imagery and Music. *Journal of the Association of Music and Imagery, 7,* 1–7.

Bruscia, K. E. (1987). *Improvisational models of music therapy.* Springfield, IL: Charles C. Thomas.

Bruscia, K. E. (1989). *Defining music therapy.* Spring City, PA: Spring House Books.

Bruscia, K. E. (Ed.). (1991). *Case studies in music therapy.* Gilsum, NH: Barcelona.

Bruscia, K. E. (1993). *Client assessment in music therapy.* Unpublished manuscript.

Bruscia, K. E. (1998a). *Defining music therapy* (2nd ed.). Gilsum, NH: Barcelona.

Bruscia, K. E. (Ed.). (1998b). *The dynamics of music psychotherapy.* Gilsum, NH: Barcelona.

Bruscia, K. E. (2001). A model of supervision derived from apprenticeship training. In M. Forinash (Ed.), *Music therapy supervision* (pp. 281–295). Gilsum, NH: Barcelona.

Bruscia, K. E. (2003, November). *Client assessment in music therapy.* Presentation at the conference of the American Music Therapy Association, St. Louis, MO.

Bruscia, K. E. (2005). Developing theory. In B. L. Wheeler (Ed.), *Music therapy research* (2nd ed.; pp. 540–551). Gilsum, NH: Barcelona.

Bruscia, K. E. (2011, November). *Ways of thinking in music therapy* (The William W. Sears Distinguished Lecture Series). Paper presented at American Music Therapy Association 13th Annual Conference, Atlanta, Georgia. Podcast retrieved from http://amtapro.musictherapy.org/?p=797

Bruscia, K. E. (2014a). *Case examples of improvisational music therapy.* Gilsum, NH: Barcelona.

Bruscia, K. E. (2014b). *Defining music therapy* (3rd ed.). University Park, IL: Barcelona.

Bruscia, K. E., & Grocke, D. E. (Eds.). (2002). *Guided Imagery and Music: The Bonny Method and beyond.* Gilsum, NH: Barcelona.

Bruscia, K. E., & Maranto, C. D. (1985, November). *The Bruscia-Maranto Projective Music Listening Test.* Paper presented at the Joint Conference on the Creative Arts Therapists, National Coalition of Arts Therapy Associations, New York, NY.

Cameron, S., & Turtle-Song, I. (2002). Learning to write case notes using the SOAP format. *Journal of Counseling and Development, 80*(3), 386–282. doi:10.1002/j.1556-6678.2002.tb00193.x

Camilleri, V. A. (2001). Therapist self-awareness: An essential tool in music therapy. *Arts in Psychotherapy, 28*(1), 79–85. doi:10.1016/S0197-4556(00)00069-1

Carpente, J. (2013). *Individual music-centered assessment profile for neurodevelopmental disorders. (IMCAP-ND): A clinical manual.* Baldwin, NY: Regina.

Carpente, J. A. (2014). Individual Music-Centered Assessment Profile for Neurodevelopmental Disorders (IMCAP-ND): New developments in music-centered evaluation. *Music Therapy Perspectives, 32*(1), 56–60. doi:10.1093/mtp/miu005

Carpente, J. A. (2016). Investigating the effectiveness of a Developmental, Individual Difference, Relationship-Based (DIR) improvisational music therapy program on social communication for children with autism spectrum disorder. *Music Therapy Perspectives.* Advance online publication. doi:10.1093/mtp/miw013

Carter, E., & Oldfield, A. (2002). A music therapy group to assist clinical diagnoses in child and family psychiatry. In A. Davies & E. Richards (Eds.), *Music therapy and group work: Sound company* (pp. 149–163). Philadelphia, PA: Jessica Kingsley.

Cartwright, C. A., & Cartwright, G. P. (1984). *Developing observation skills* (2ⁿᵈ ed.). New York, NY: McGraw-Hill.

Cassity, M. D. (1976). The influence of a music therapy activity upon peer acceptance, group cohesiveness, and interpersonal relationships of adult psychiatric patients. *Journal of Music Therapy, 13*(2), 66–76. doi:10.1093/jmt/13.2.66

Cassity, M. D., & Cassity, J. E. (2006). *Multimodal psychiatric music therapy for adults, adolescents, and children* (3ʳᵈ ed.). London, UK: Jessica Kingsley.

Cattell, R. B., & Anderson, J. C. (1953). The measurement of personality and behavior disorders by the IPAT Music Preference Test. *Journal of Applied Psychology, 37*(6), 446–454. doi:10.1037/h0056224

Cattell, R. B., & McMichael, R. E. (1960). Clinical diagnosis by the IPAT Music Preference Test. *Journal of Consulting Psychology, 24*(4), 333–341. doi:10.1037/h0044418

Certification Board for Music Therapists. (2011). *Code of Professional Practice.* Retrieved from www.cbmt.org/about-certification/code-of-professional-practice/

Certification Board for Music Therapists. (2015a). *Board Certification Domains.* Retrieved from www.cbmt.org/

Certification Board for Music Therapists. (2015b). American Music Therapy Association. *Scope of Music Therapy Practice.* Retrieved from www.cbmt.org/; www.musictherapy.org/about/scope_of_music_therapy_practice/ (home; Scope of Music Therapy Practice).

Cevasco, A. (2014). Music technology in the neonatal intensive care unit. In W. L. Magee (Ed.), *Music technology in therapeutic and health settings* (pp. 111–132). London, UK: Jessica Kingsley.

Chase, K. M. (2002). *The music therapy assessment handbook.* Columbus, MS: Southern Pen.

Chase, M. P. (1974). *Just being at the piano.* Culver City, CA: Peace Press.

Chavin, M. (1991). *The lost chord.* Mt. Airy, MD: ElderSong.

Chlan, L., & Heiderscheit, A. (2009). A tool for music preference assessment in critically ill patients receiving mechanical ventilatory support. *Music Therapy Perspectives, 27*(1), 42–47. doi:10.1093/mtp/27.1.42

Choi, B. (2008). Awareness of music therapy practices and factors influencing specific theoretical approaches. *Journal of Music Therapy, 45*(1), 93–109. doi:10.1093/jmt/45.1.93

Clair, A., & Memmott, J. (2008). *Therapeutic uses of music* with older adults (2nd ed.). Silver Spring, MD: American Music Therapy Association.

Clair, A. A. (1996). *Therapeutic uses of music with older adults.* Baltimore, MD: Health Professions Press.

Clark, C., & Chadwick, D. (1979). *Clinically adapted instruments for the multiply handicapped.* St. Louis, MO: Magnamusic-Baton.

Clements-Cortes, A. (2015). A survey study of pre-professionals' understanding of the Canadian music therapy internship experience. *Journal of Music Therapy, 52*(2), 221–257. doi:10.1093/jmt/thv006

Clements-Cortes, A., Ahonen, H., Evans, M., Freedman, M., & Bartell, L. (2016). Short-term effects of rhythmic sensory stimulation in Alzheimer's disease: An exploratory pilot study. *Journal of Alzheimer's Disease, 52*(2), 651–660. doi:10.3233/JAD-160081

Cohen, G., & Gericke, O. L. (1972). Music therapy assessment: Prime requisite for determining patient objectives. *Journal of Music Therapy, 9*(4), 161–189. doi:10.1093/jmt/9.4.161

Coleman, K., & Brunk, B. (1997). *Prelude: Music therapy assessment kit: Special education edition* (1997 revision). Grapevine, TX: Prelude Music Therapy.

Coleman, K. A., & Brunk, B. K. (2003). *SEMTAP: Special Education Music Therapy Assessment Process handbook* (2nd ed.). Grapevine, TX: Prelude Music Therapy.

Come Join the Geritones. (n.d.). Lake Forest, IL: The Geri-Tones.

Cordrey, C. (1994). *Hidden treasures: Music and memory activities for people with Alzheimer's.* Mt. Airy, MD: ElderSong.

Corey, G. (2009). *Theory and practice of counseling and psychotherapy* (8th ed.). Belmont, CA: Brooks/Cole.

Corey, G., Corey, M. S., Callanan, P., & Russell, J. M. (2014). *Group techniques* (4th ed.). Pacific Grove, CA: Brooks/Cole.

Corey, G., Corey, M. S., Corey, C., & Callanan, P. (2014). *Issues and ethics in the helping professions* (9th ed.). Boston, MA: Cengage.

Corey, M. S., & Corey, G. (2015). *Becoming a helper* (7th ed.). Boston, MA: Cengage.

Corsini, R. J., & Wedding, D. (2007). *Current psychotherapies* (8th ed.). Belmont, CA: Brooks/Cole.

Cozolino, L. (2004). *The making of a therapist: A practical guide to the inner journey.* New York, NY: W. W. Norton Co.

Critchley, M. (1977). Musicogenic epilepsy. I. The beginnings. In M. Critchley & R. Henson (Eds.), *Music and the brain* (pp. 344–353). London, UK: William Heineman Medical Books Ltd.

Darnley-Smith, R., & Patey, H. M. (2003). *Music therapy.* London, UK: Sage.

Darrow, A-A. (2008). *Introduction to approaches in music therapy* (2nd ed.). Silver Spring, MD: American Music Therapy Association.

Dass, R., & Gorman, P. (1985). *How can I help? Stories and reflections on service.* New York, NY: Alfred A. Knopf.

Dassa, A., & Amir, D. (2014). The role of singing familiar songs in encouraging conversation among people with middle to late-stage Alzheimer's disease. *Journal of Music Therapy, 51*(2), 131–153. doi:10.1093/jmt/thu007

Davies, A., & Richards, E. (2002). *Music therapy and group work: Sound company.* London, UK: Jessica Kingsley.

Davies, A., Richards, E., & Barwick, N. (2014). *Group music therapy: A group analytic approach.* East Sussex, UK: Routledge.

De Backer, J., & Van Camp, J. (1999). Specific aspects of the music therapy relationship to psychiatry. In T. Wigram & J. De Backer (Eds.), *Clinical applications of music therapy in psychiatry* (pp. 11–23). Philadelphia, PA: Jessica Kingsley.

Deschênes, B. (1995). Music and symbols. *Music Therapy Perspectives, 13*(1), 40–45. doi:10.1093/mtp/13.1.40

Dileo, C. (1999). (Ed.). *Music therapy & medicine: Theoretical and clinical applications.* Silver Spring, MD: American Music Therapy Association.

Dileo, C. (2000). *Ethical thinking in music therapy.* Cherry Hill, NJ: Jeffrey Books.

Dileo, C., & Bradt, J. (1999). Entrainment, resonance, and pain-related suffering. In C. Dileo (Ed.), *Music therapy and medicine: Theoretical and clinical applications* (pp. 181–188). Silver Spring, MD: American Music Therapy Association.

Dobson, K. (Ed.). (1988). *Handbook of cognitive-behavioral therapies.* New York, NY: Guilford Press.

Dolan, Y. (1991*). Resolving sexual abuse: Solutions-focused therapy and Ericksonian hypnosis for adult survivors.* New York, NY: Norton.

Doran, G. T. (1981). There's a S.M.A.R.T. way to write management's goals and objectives. *Management Review, 70*(11), 35–36.

Dosman, C. F., Andrews, D., & Goulden, K. J. (2012). Evidence-based milestone ages as a framework for developmental surveillance. *Paediatric Child Health, 17*(10), 561–568.

Dvorkin, J. (1998). Transference and countertransference in group improvisation therapy. In K. E. Bruscia (Ed.), *The dynamics of music psychotherapy* (pp. 287–298). Gilsum, NH: Barcelona.

Egan, G. (1975). *The skilled helper: A model for systematic helping and interpersonal relating.* Monterey, CA: Brooks/Cole.

Erikson, E. (1963). *Childhood and society* (2nd ed.). New York, NY: W. W. Norton & Co. (Original work published 1950)

Eschen, J. T. (Ed.). (2002). *Analytical Music Therapy.* Philadelphia, PA: Jessica Kingsley.

Eyre, L. (2011a). From ego disintegration to recovery of self: The contribution of Lacan's theories in understanding the role of music therapy in the treatment of a woman with psychosis. In A. Meadows (Ed.), *Developments in music therapy practice: Case study examples* (pp. 385–399). Gilsum, NH: Barcelona.

Eyre, L. (2011b). Therapeutic chorale for persons with chronic mental illness: A descriptive survey of participant experiences. *Journal of Music Therapy, 48*(2), 149–168. doi:10.1093/jmt/48.2.149

Eyre, L. (2013). Adult groups in the inpatient setting. In L. Eyre (Ed.), *Guidelines for music therapy practice in mental health* (pp. 71–114). University Park, IL: Barcelona.

Farnan, L., & Johnson, F. (1988a). *Everyone can move.* New Berlin, WI: Jenson.

Farnan, L., & Johnson, F. (1988b). *Music is for everyone.* New Berlin, WI: Jenson.

Feil, N. (1980). *Validation fantasy therapy: VF, the Feil Method.* Cleveland, OH: Author.

Feil, N. (2002). *The validation breakthrough: Simple techniques for communicating with people with Alzheimer's-type dementia.* Towson, MD: Health Professions Press.

Feil, N. (2008). Validation Therapy. In E. Capezuli, E. L. Siegler, & M. Mezey (Eds.), *Encyclopedia of elder care* (2nd ed., pp. 797–799). New York, NY: Springer.

Fischer, R. (1991). Original song drawings in the treatment of a developmentally disabled, autistic adult. In K. E. Bruscia (Ed.), *Case studies in music therapy* (pp. 359–371). Gilsum, NH: Barcelona.

Forinash, M. (2001). *Music therapy supervision.* Gilsum, NH: Barcelona.

Frank, J. D., & Frank, J. B. (1991). *Persuasion and healing: A comparative study of psychiatry* (3rd ed.). Baltimore, MD: Johns Hopkins University Press.

Freud, S. (1938). *The basic writings of Sigmund Freud* (A. A. Brill, trans.). New York, NY: Random House.

Frohne-Hagemann, I. (Ed.), (2007). *Receptive music therapy*. Wiesbaden, Germany: Zeitpunkt Musik.

Gagné, R. M., & Briggs, L. J. (1974). *Principles of instructional design* (2nd ed.). New York, NY: Holt, Rinehart, and Winston.

Gallagher, L. M., & Steele, A. L. (2002). Music therapy with offenders in a substance abuse/mental illness treatment program. *Music Therapy Perspectives, 20*(2), 117–122. doi:10.1093/mtp/20.2.117

Gardstrom, S. C. (2007). *Music therapy improvisation for groups: Essential leadership competencies*. Gilsum, NH: Barcelona.

Gardstrom, S. C., & Jackson, N. A. (2011). Personal therapy for undergraduate music therapy students: A survey of AMTA program coordinators. *Journal of Music Therapy, 48*(2), 226–255. doi:10.1093/jmt/48.2.226

Garland, J., Jones, H., & Kolodny, R. L. (1976). A model for stages of development in social work groups. In S. Bernstein (Ed.), *Explorations in group work: Essays in theory and practice* (pp. 17–71). Boston, MA: Charles River Books.

Garrett, P., & Seidman, J. (2011, January 24). EMR vs. EHR—What is the difference? (Blog post). Retrieved from www.healthit.gov/buzz-blog/electronic-health-and-medical-records/emr-vs-ehr-difference/

Gehart, D. R. (2014). *Mastering competencies in family therapy: A practical approach to theory and clinical case documentation* (2nd ed.). Belmont, CA: Brooks/Cole.

Gfeller, K. (1987). Songwriting as a tool for reading and language remediation. *Music Therapy, 6*(2), 28–38. doi:10.1093/mt/6.2.28

Gfeller, K., & Hanson, N. (1995). *Music therapy programming for individuals with Alzheimer's disease and related disorders*. Iowa City, IA: University of Iowa.

Ghetti, C., & Hannan, A. (2008). Pediatric intensive care unit (PICU). In D. Hanson-Abromeit & C. Colwell (Eds.), *Medical music therapy for pediatrics in hospital settings* (pp. 71–106). Silver Spring, MD: American Music Therapy Association.

Gill-Thwaites, H., & Munday, R. (2004). The sensory modality assessment and rehabilitation techniques (SMART): A valid and reliable assessment for vegetative state and minimally conscious state patients. *Brain Injury, 18*(12), 1255–1269. doi:10.1080/02699050410001719952

Glassman, L. R. (1983). The talent show: Meeting the needs of the healthy elderly. *Music Therapy, 3*(1), 82–93. doi:10.1093/mt/3.1.82

Goldfried, M. R. (2001). *How therapists change: Personal and professional reflections*. Washington, DC: American Psychological Association.

Gooding, L., & Standley, J. (2011). Musical development and learning characteristics of students: A compilation of key points from the research literature organized by age. *Update: Applications of Research in Music Education, 30*(1), 32–45. doi:10.1177/8755123311418481

Goodman, K. D. (1989). Music therapy assessment of emotionally disturbed children. *Arts in Psychotherapy, 16*(3), 179–192. doi:10.1016/0197-4556(89)90021-X

Goodman, K. D. (2007). *Music therapy groupwork with special needs children*. Springfield, IL: Charles C. Thomas.

Graham, M. E. (2016). Toward a practice of engaged filming in Nordoff-Robbins Music Therapy. *Music Therapy Perspectives, 34*(1), 64–70. doi:10.1093/mtp/miu052

Grant, R. (1973). *Sing along, senior citizens.* Springfield, IL: Charles C. Thomas.

Grant, R. E., & McCarty, B. (1990). Emotional stages in the music therapy internship. *Journal of Music Therapy, 27*(3), 102–118. doi:10.1093/jmt/27.3.102

Greenspan, S. I. (1992*). Infancy and early childhood: The practice of clinical assessment and intervention with emotional and developmental challenges.* Madison, CT: International Universities Press.

Greenspan, S. I., & Wieder, S. (1998). *The child with special needs: Encouraging intellectual and emotional growth.* Reading, MA: Addison-Wesley.

Grocke, D., & Wigram, T. (2007). *Receptive methods in music therapy.* London, UK: Jessica Kingsley.

Gustorff, D. (2001). Beyond words: Music therapy with comatose patients and those with impaired consciousness in intensive care. In D. Aldridge, G. DiFranco, E. Ruud, & T. Wigram (Eds.), *Music therapy in Europe* (pp. 61–72). Rome, Italy: ISMEZ.

Hadley, S. (1996). A rationale for the use of songs with children undergoing bone marrow transplantation. *Australian Journal of Music Therapy, 7,* 16–27.

Hadley, S. (Ed.). (2003). *Psychodynamic music therapy: Case studies.* Gilsum, NH: Barcelona.

Hadley, S., & Yancy, G. (Eds.). (2012). *Therapeutic uses of rap and hip-hop.* New York, NY: Routledge.

Hadsell, N. A. (1993). Levels of external structure in music therapy. *Music Therapy Perspectives, 11*(2), 61–65. doi:10.1093/mtp/11.2.61

Hall, R. V., & Van Houten, R. (1983). *Managing behavior 1: Behavior modification: The measurement of behavior.* Austin, TX: Pro-Ed.

Hanser, S. B. (1990). A music therapy strategy for depressed older adults in the community. *Journal of Applied Gerontology, 9*(3), 283–298. doi:10.1177/073346489000900304

Hanser, S. B. (1999). *The new music therapist's handbook* (2nd ed.). Boston, MA: Berklee Press.

Hanser, S. B. (2016). *Integrative health through music therapy.* New York, NY: MacMillan.

Hanser, S. B., & Thompson, L. W. (1994). Effects of a music therapy strategy on depressed older adults. *Journal of Gerontology: Psychological Sciences, 49*(6), 265–269. doi:10.1093/geronj/49.6.P265

Hanson-Abromeit, D., & Colwell, C. (Eds.). (2008). *Medical music therapy for pediatrics in hospital settings.* Silver Spring, MD: American Music Therapy Association.

Hanson-Abromeit, D., & Colwell, C. (Eds.). (2010). *Medical music therapy for adults in hospital settings.* Silver Spring, MD: American Music Therapy Association.

Heimlich, E. P. (1965). The specialized use of music as a mode of communication in the treatment of disturbed children. *Journal of the American Academy of Child Psychiatry, 4*(1), 86–122. doi:10.1016/S0002-7138(09)62072-0

Heimlich, E. P. (1972). Paraverbal techniques in the therapy of childhood communication disorders. *International Journal of Child Psychotherapy, 1,* 65–83.

Herman, F. (1991). The boy that nobody wanted: Creative experiences for a boy with severe emotional problems. In K. E. Bruscia (Ed.), *Case studies in music therapy* (pp. 99–108). Gilsum, NH: Barcelona.

Hertrampf, R., & Klinken, H. S. (2015). Group Music and Imagery (GrpMI) therapy with female cancer patients. In D. Grocke & T. Moe (Eds.), *Guided Imagery and Music (GIM) and music imagery methods for individual and group therapy* (pp. 243–251). London, UK: Jessica Kingsley.

Hesser, B. (2001). The transformative power of music in our lives: A personal perspective. *Music Therapy Perspectives, 19*(1), 53–58. doi:10.1093/mtp/19.1.53

Hibben, J. (1991). Group music therapy with a classroom of 6–8-year-old hyperactive-learning disabled children. In K. E. Bruscia (Ed.), *Case studies in music therapy* (pp. 175–189). Gilsum, NH: Barcelona.

Hibben, J. (Ed.). (1999). *Inside music therapy: Client experiences.* Gilsum, NH: Barcelona.

Hintz, M. (2000). Geriatric music therapy clinical assessment: Assessment of music skills and related behaviors. *Music Therapy Perspectives, 18*(1), 31–40. doi:10.1093/mtp/18.1.31

Hintz, M. R. (2013a). Autism. In M. R. Hintz (Ed.), *Guidelines for music therapy practice in developmental health* (pp. 50–86). Gilsum, NH: Barcelona.

Hintz, M. R. (Ed.). (2013b). *Guidelines for music therapy practice in developmental health.* Gilsum, NH: Barcelona.

Hoffren, J. (1964). A test of musical expression. *Bulletin of the Council for Research in Music Education, 2,* 32–35.

Hong, S., & Choi, M. J. (2011). Songwriting-oriented activities improve the cognitive functions of the aged with dementia. *Arts in Psychotherapy, 38*(4), 221–228. doi:10.1016/j.aip.2011.07.002

Horikoshi, T., Asari, Y., Watanabe, A., Nagaseki, Y., Nukui, H., Sasaki, H., & Komiya, K. (1997). Music alexia in a patient with mild pure alexia: Distorted visual perception of nonverbal meaningful figures. *Cortex, 33*(1), 187–194. doi:10.1016/S0010-9452(97)80014-7

Hough, S. (1982). The nature of musical communication, group interaction, and social independence among preschool children. Unpublished master's thesis, Southern Methodist University, Dallas, TX.

Humphries, C. (2010). *The piano improvisation handbook.* Milwaukee, WI: Hal Leonard.

Hurt, C. P., Rice, R. R., McIntosh, G. C., & Thaut, M. H. (1998). Rhythmic Auditory Stimulation in gait training for patients with traumatic brain injury. *Journal of Music Therapy, 35*(4), 228–241. doi:10.1093/jmt/35.4.228

Hurt-Thaut, C. P., & Johnson, S. B. (2015). In B. L. Wheeler (Ed.), *Music therapy handbook* (pp. 220–232). New York, NY: Guilford Press.

Husni-Palacios, M., & Palacios, J. R. (1964). Auditory perception and personality patterns in blind adults. *Journal of Projective Techniques and Personality Assessment, 28*(3), 284–292. doi:10.1080/0091651X.1964.10120135

"Identity." (2016). In *Merriam-Webster online dictionary*. Retrieved from www.merriam-webster.com/dictionary/identity

Ivey, A. E., Ivey, M. B., & Zalaquett, C. P. (2014). *Intentional interviewing and counseling: Facilitating client development in a multicultural society* (8th ed.). Boston, MA: Cengage.

Ivey, A. E., & Simek-Downing, L. (1980). *Counseling and psychotherapy: Skills, theories, and practice.* Englewood Cliffs, NJ: Prentice-Hall.

Jacobsen, S. (2012). Music therapy assessment and development of parental competences in families with children who have experienced emotional neglect: An investigation of the reliability and validity of the tool, Assessment of Parenting Competencies (APC). Unpublished PhD Dissertation, Aalborg University, Aalborg, Denmark. Retrieved from http://www.mt-phd.aau.dk/phd-theses/

Jacobsen, S., & Wigram, T. (2007). Music therapy for the Assessment of Parental Competencies for children in need of care. *Nordic Journal of Music Therapy, 16*(2), 129–143. doi:10.1080/08098130709478182

Jacobsen, S. L., & McKinney, C. H. (2015). A music therapy tool for assessing parent–child interaction in cases of emotional neglect. *Journal of Child and Family Studies, 24*(7), 2164–2173. doi:10.1007/s10826-014-0019-0

James, M. R., & Freed, B. S. (1989). A sequential model for developing group cohesion in music therapy. *Music Therapy Perspectives, 7*(1), 28–34. doi:10.1093/mtp/7.1.28

"Jazzy," Hunter, L. L., & Polen, D. W. (1999). Jazzy the Wonder Squirrel. In J. Hibben (Ed.), *Inside music therapy: Client experiences* (pp. 87–95). Gilsum, NH: Barcelona.

Jeong, E. (2013). Psychometric validation of a music-based attention assessment: revised for patients with traumatic brain injury. *Journal of Music Therapy, 50*(2), 66–92. doi:10.1093/jmt/50.2.66

Jeong, E., & Lesiuk, T. L. (2011). Development and preliminary evaluation of a Music-Based Attention Assessment for patients with traumatic brain injury. *Journal of Music Therapy, 48*(4), 551–572. doi:10.1093/jmt/48.4.55

Jordan, J. (1999). *The musician's soul.* Chicago, IL: GIA.

Katagiri, J. (2009). The effect of background music and song texts on the emotional understanding of children with autism. *Journal of Music Therapy, 45*(1), 15–31. doi:10.1093/jmt/46.1.15

Katsh, S., & Merle-Fishman, C. (1998). *The music within you* (2nd ed.). Gilsum, NH: Barcelona.

Kenny, C. (2006). *Music and life in the Field of Play: An anthology.* Gilsum, NH: Barcelona.

Kenny, C. B. (1985). Music: A whole systems approach. *Music Therapy, 5*(1), 3–11. doi:10.1093/mt/5.1.3

Kenny, C. B. (1989). *The Field of Play: A guide for the theory and practice of music therapy.* Atascadero, CA: Ridgeview.

Keough, L. A., King, B., & Lemmerman, T. (2016). Assessment-based small-group music therapy programming for individuals with dementia and Alzheimer's disease: A multiyear clinical project. *Music Therapy Perspectives.* Advance online publication. doi:10.1093/mtp/miw021

Kern, P. (2012). Resources within reach: information at your fingertips. In P. Kern & M. Humpal (Eds.), *Early childhood music therapy and autism spectrum disorders: Developing potential in young children and their families* (pp. 265–279). London, UK: Jessica Kingsley.

Klein, R. H., Bernard, H. S., & Schermer, V. L. (2011). *On becoming a psychotherapist: The personal and professional journey.* New York, NY: Oxford University Press.

Knight, A., & LaGasse, A. B. (2012). Reconnecting to music technology: Looking back and looking forward. *Music Therapy Perspectives, 30*(2), 188–195. doi:10.1093/mtp/30.2.188

Knight, A. J. (2008). Music therapy internship supervisors and pre-internship students: A comparative analysis of questionnaires. *Journal of Music Therapy, 45*(1), 75–92. doi:10.1093/jmt/45.1.75

Kramer, C. H. (2000). *Therapeutic mastery: Becoming a more creative and effective therapist.* Phoenix, AZ: Zeig, Tucker, & Co., Inc.

Krout, R. E. (2016). Measurement of clinical events and processes. In B. L. Wheeler & K. M. Murphy (Eds.), *Music therapy research* (3rd ed., pp. 169–181). University Park, IL: Barcelona.

Lane, D. (1991). The effect of a single music therapy session on hospitalized children as measured by salivary immunoglobulin a, speech pause time, and patient opinion Likert scale. *Pediatric Research, 29*(Pt. 2), 119–125.

Layman, D. L., Hussey, D. L., & Laing, S. J. (2002). Music therapy assessment for severely emotionally disturbed children: A pilot study. *Journal of Music Therapy, 39*(3), 164–187. doi:10.1093/jmt/39.3.164

Layman, D. L., Hussey, D. L., & Reed, A. M. (2013). The Beech Brook group treatment assessment tool: A pilot study. *Journal of Music Therapy, 50*(3), 155–175. doi:10.1093/jmt/50.3.155

Lazarus, A. A. (1976). *Multimodal behavior therapy.* New York, NY: Springer.

Lazarus, A. A. (1989). *The practice of multimodal therapy.* Baltimore, MD: John Hopkins University Press.

Ledger, A., & Baker, F. (2007). An investigation of long-term effects of group music therapy on agitation levels of people with Alzheimer's disease. *Aging & Mental Health, 11*(3), 330–338. doi:10.1080/13607860600963406

Lee, C., & Houde, M. (2010). *Improvising in styles: A workbook for music therapists, educators, and musicians.* Gilsum, NH: Barcelona.

Leepeng, P. T. (2004). The effects of background music on quality of sleep in elementary school children. *Journal of Music Therapy, 41*(2), 128–150. doi:10.1093/jmt/41.2.128.

Levin, H., & Levin, G. (1977). *A garden of bell flowers.* Bryn Mawr, PA: Theodore Presser.

Levin, H., & Levin, G. (1997). *Learning through songs.* Gilsum, NH: Barcelona.

Levin, H., & Levin, G. (1998). *Learning through music.* Gilsum, NH: Barcelona.

Levin, H., & Levin, G. (2004). *Distant bells: 12 delightful melodies from distant lands arranged for resonator bells & piano.* Gilsum, NH: Barcelona.

Liberatore, A. M., & Layman, D. L. (1999). *The Cleveland Music Therapy Assessment of Infants and Toddlers: A practical guide to assessment and developing intervention.* Cleveland, OH: Cleveland Music School Settlement.

Lipe, A. W. (2015). Music therapy assessment. In B. L. Wheeler (Ed.), *Music therapy handbook* (pp. 76–90). New York, NY: Guilford Press.

Loewy, J. (1999). The use of music psychotherapy in the treatment of pediatric pain. In C. Dileo (Ed.), *Music therapy and medicine: Theoretical and clinical applications* (pp. 189–206). Silver Spring, MD: American Music Therapy Association.

Loewy, J. (2000). Music psychotherapy assessment. *Music Therapy Perspectives, 18*(1), 47–58. doi:10.1093/mtp/18.1.47

Loewy, J., MacGregor, B., Richards, K., & Rodriguez, J. (1997). Music therapy in pediatric pain management: Attending to the sounds of hurt, fear, and anxiety. In J. Loewy (Ed.), *Music therapy and pediatric pain* (pp. 45–56). Cherry Hill, NJ: Jeffrey Books.

Madsen, C. H., Jr., & Madsen, C. K. (1983). *Teaching/discipline: A positive approach for educational development* (3rd ed.). Raleigh, NC: Contemporary.

Madsen, C. K. (1980). *Behavior modification and music therapy: A guide for working with the mentally retarded.* Washington, DC: National Association for Music Therapy.

Madsen, C. K., & Kaiser, K. A. (1999). Pre-internship fears of music therapists. *Journal of Music Therapy, 36*(1), 17–25. doi:10.1093/jmt/36.1.17

Magee, W. (1999). "Singing my life, playing my self": Song-based and improvisatory methods of music therapy with individuals with neurological impairments. In T. Wigram & J. De Backer (Eds.), *Clinical applications of music therapy in developmental disability, paediatrics, and neurology* (pp. 201–223). London, UK: Jessica Kingsley.

Magee, W. L. (Ed.). (2014). *Music technology in therapeutic and health settings.* London, UK: Jessica Kingsley.

Magee, W. L., Bertolami, M. A., Kubicek, L., LaJoie, M., Martino, L., Sankowski, A., Townsend, J., Whitehead-Pleaux, A. M., & Zigo, J. B. (2011). Using music technology in music therapy with populations across the life span in medical and educational programs. *Music and Medicine, 3*(3), 146–153. doi:10.1177/1943862111403005

Magee, W. L., Ghetti, C. M., & Moyer, A. (2015). Feasibility of the music therapy assessment tool for awareness in disorders of consciousness (MATADOC) for use with pediatric populations. *Frontiers of Psychology, 6,* 698. doi:10.3389/fpsyg.2015.00698

Magee, W. L., Siegert, R. J., Daveson, B. A., Lenton-Smith, G., & Taylor, S. M. (2014). Music therapy assessment tool for awareness in disorders of consciousness (MATADOC): Standardisation of the principal subscale to assess awareness in patients with disorders of consciousness. *Neuropsychology Rehabilitation, 24*(1), 101–124. doi:10.1080/09602011.2013.844174

Magee, W. L., Siegert, R. J., Taylor, S. M., Daveson, B. A., & Lenton-Smith, G. (2016). Music therapy assessment tool for awareness in disorders of consciousness (MATADOC): Reliability and validity of a measure to assess awareness in patients with disorders of consciousness. *Journal of Music Therapy, 53*(1), 1–26. doi:10.1093/jmt/thv017

Maranto, C. D. (Ed.). (1993). *Music therapy: International perspectives.* Pipersville, PA: Jeffrey Books.

Marley, L. (1996). Music therapy with hospitalized infants and toddlers in a child life program. In M. A. R. Froelich (Ed.), *Music therapy with hospitalized children* (pp. 77–86). Cherry Hill, NJ: Jeffrey Books.

Marsalis, W. (2008). *Moving to higher ground: How jazz can change your life.* New York, NY: Random House.

Martin, L. K. (2012). Applied behavior analysis: Introduction and practical application in music therapy for young children with autism spectrum disorders. In P. Kern & M. Humpal (Eds.), *Early childhood music therapy and autism spectrum disorders: Developing potential in young children and their families* (pp. 101–116). London, UK: Jessica Kingsley.

Maslow, A. H. (1999). *Toward a psychology of being* (3rd ed.). New York, NY: John Wiley & Sons.

Matthews, G., Jones, D. M., & Chamberlain, A. G. (1990). Refining the measurement of mood: The UWIST Mood Adjective Check List. *British Journal of Psychology, 81*(1), 17–42. doi:10.1111/j.2044-8295.1990.tb02343.x

Mazzagatti, N. (1975). The Mazzagatti Auditory Perception Technique (MAAT). *The New Jersey Psychologist, 26*(1), 10–12.

McDermott, O., Orrell, M., & Ridder, H. M. (2015). The development of Music in Dementia Assessment Scales (MiDAS). *Nordic Journal of Music Therapy, 24*(3), 232–251. doi:10.1080/08098131.2014.907333

McDonnell, L. (1983). Music therapy: Meeting the psychosocial needs of hospitalized children. *Journal of the Association for the Care of Children's Health, 12*(1), 29–33.

McFerran, K. (2010). *Adolescents, music and music therapy: Methods and techniques for clinicians, educators and students.* London, UK: Jessica Kingsley.

McFerran, K. (2016). How music can change your life ... and the world. *Voices: A World Forum for Music Therapy, 16*(2). Retrieved from https://voices.no/index.php/voices/article/view/886/728. doi:10.15845/voices.v16i2.886

McFerran, K., & Teggelove, K. (2011). Music therapy with young people in schools: After the Black Saturday fires. *Voices: A World Forum for Music Therapy, 11*(1). Retrieved from

https://voices.no/index.php/voices/article/view/285.
doi:10.15845/voices.v11i1.285

McGuire, M. G., & Smeltekop, R. A. (1994a). The termination process in music therapy: Part I—Theory and clinical implementations. *Music Therapy Perspectives, 12*(1), 20–27. doi:10.1093/mtp/12.1.20

McGuire, M. G., & Smeltekop, R. A. (1994b). The termination process in music therapy: Part II—A model and clinical applications. *Music Therapy Perspectives, 12*(1), 28–34. doi:10.1093/mtp/12.1.28

McLaughlin, B., & Adler, R. F. (2015). Music therapy for children with intellectual disabilities. In B. L. Wheeler (Ed.), *Music therapy handbook* (pp. 277–289). New York: NY: Guilford Press.

Meadows, A. (2000). The validity and reliability of the Guided Imagery and Music Responsiveness Scale. *Journal of the Association for Music and Imagery, 7,* 8–33.

Meadows, A. (Ed.). (2011). *Developments in music therapy practice: Case study perspectives.* Gilsum, NH: Barcelona.

Meadows, A. (2015). Music and imagery in cancer care. In D. Grocke & T. Moe (Eds.), *Guided Imagery and Music (GIM) and music imagery methods for individual and group therapy* (pp. 189–197). London, UK: Jessica Kingsley.

Medley, D. M. (1982). Systematic observation. In H. E. Mitzel (Ed.), *Encyclopedia of educational research* (5th ed., pp. 1841–1851). New York, NY: Free Press.

Merle-Fishman, C. R., & Marcus, M. L. (1982). Musical behaviors and preferences of emotionally disturbed and normal children: An exploratory study. *Music Therapy, 2*(1), 1–11. doi:10.1093/mt/2.1.1

Murphy, K. M. (2015). Music therapy in addictions treatment. In B. L. Wheeler (Ed.), *Music therapy handbook* (pp. 354–366). New York, NY: Guilford Press.

Murphy, K. M., & Wheeler, B. L. (2005). Symposium on experiential learning in music therapy: Report of the symposium sponsored by the World Federation of Music Therapy Commission on Education, Training, and Accreditation. *Music Therapy Perspectives, 23*(2), 138–143. doi:10.1093/mtp/23.2.138

Murphy, M. (1983). Music therapy: A self-help group experience for substance abuse patients. *Music Therapy, 3*(1), 52–62. doi:10.1093/mt/3.1.52

Naghdi, L., Ahonen, A., Macario, P., & Bartel, L. (2015). The effect of low-frequency sound stimulation on patients with fibromyalgia: A clinical study. *Pain Research and Management, 20*(1), 21–27. doi:10.1155/2015/375174

Nicholson, J. M., Berthelsen, D., Abad, V., Williams, K., & Bradley, J. (2008). Impact of music therapy to promote positive parenting and child development. *Journal of Health Psychology, 13*(2), 226–238. doi:10.1177/1359105307086705J

Nordoff, P., & Robbins, C. (1962). *The first book of children's play songs.* Bryn Mawr, PA: Theodore Presser.

Nordoff, P., & Robbins, C. (1966). *The three bears.* Bryn Mawr, PA: Theodore Presser.

Nordoff, P., & Robbins, C. (1968a). *Fun for four drums.* Bryn Mawr, PA: Theodore Presser.

Nordoff, P., & Robbins, C. (1968b). *The second book of children's play songs.* Bryn Mawr, PA: Theodore Presser.

Nordoff, P., & Robbins, C. (1969). *Pif-paf-poltrie.* Bryn Mawr, PA: Theodore Presser.

Nordoff, P., & Robbins, C. (1971). *Therapy in music for handicapped children.* New York, NY: St. Martin's Press.

Nordoff, P., & Robbins, C. (1972). *Spirituals.* Bryn Mawr, PA: Theodore Presser.

Nordoff, P., & Robbins, C. (1979). *Fanfares and dances.* Bryn Mawr, PA: Theodore Presser.

Nordoff, P., & Robbins, C. (1980a). *The third book of children's play songs.* Bryn Mawr, PA: Theodore Presser.

Nordoff, P., & Robbins, C. (1980b). *The fourth book of children's play songs.* Bryn Mawr, PA: Theodore Presser.

Nordoff, P., & Robbins, C. (1980c). *The fifth book of children's play songs.* Bryn Mawr, PA: Theodore Presser.

Nordoff, P., & Robbins, C. (1983). *Music therapy in special education* (2nd ed.). St. Louis, MO: MMB Music.

Nordoff, P., & Robbins, C. (1995). *Greetings and good-byes.* Bryn Mawr, PA: Theodore Presser.

Nordoff, P., & Robbins, C. (2007). *Creative Music Therapy: A guide to fostering clinical musicianship.* University Park, IL: Barcelona.

Norman, R. (2012). Music therapy assessment of older adults in nursing homes. *Music Therapy Perspectives, 30*(1), 8–16. doi:10.1093/mtp/30.1.8

O'Brien, E. (2006). Opera therapy: Creating and performing a new work with cancer patients and professional singers. *Nordic Journal of Music Therapy, 15*(1), 82–96. doi:10.1080/08098130609478153

O'Callaghan, C. (2005). Song writing in threatened lives. In J. V. Loewy & C. Dileo (Eds.), *Music therapy at the end of life* (pp. 117–127). Cherry Hill, NJ: Jeffrey Books.

Odell-Miller, H., & Richards, E. (2009). *Supervision of music therapy: A theoretical and practical handbook.* London, UK: Routledge.

Okun, B. F., & Kantrowitz, R. E. (2015). *Effective helping: Interviewing and counseling techniques* (8th ed.). Boston, MA: Cengage.

Oldfield, A., & Bunce, L. (2001). "Mummy can play too ..." Short-term music therapy with mothers and young children. *British Journal of Music Therapy, 15*(1), 27–36.

Parvaiz, M. A., Subramanian, A., & Kendall, N. S. (2008). The use of abbreviations in medical records in a multidisciplinary world—An imminent disaster. *Communication and Medicine, 5*(1), 25–33. doi:10.1558/cam.v5i1.25

Pattison, P. (1991). *Songwriting: Essential guide to lyric form and structure.* Boston, MA: Berklee Press.

Pavlicevic, M. (2003). *Groups in music: Strategies from music therapy.* London, UK: Jessica Kingsley.

Pavlicevic, M., & Ansdell, G. (Eds.). (2004). *Community Music Therapy.* London, UK: Jessica Kingsley.

Pavlicevic, M., & Trevarthen, C. (1989). A musical assessment of psychiatric states in adults. *Psychopathology, 22*(6), 325–334. doi:10.1159/000284615

Pennebaker, J. W. (1997). *Opening up: The healing power of expressing emotions* (2nd ed.). New York, NY: Guilford Press.

Persoons, J., & De Backer, J. (1997). Vibroacoustic music therapy with handicapped and autistic adolescents. In T. Wigram & C. Dileo (Eds.), *Music vibration* (pp. 143–148). Cherry Hill, NJ: Jeffrey Books.

Plach, T. (1980). *The creative use of music in group therapy.* Springfield, IL: Charles C. Thomas.

Polen, D. W. (1985). *Music therapy assessment for adults with developmental disabilities.* Unpublished manuscript.

Pothoulaki, M., MacDonald, R., & Flowers, P. (2012). An interpretative phenomenological analysis of an improvisational music therapy program for cancer patients. *Journal of Music Therapy, 49*(1), 45–67. doi:10.1093/jmt/49.1.45

Priestley, M. (1975). *Music therapy in action.* London, UK: Constable.

Priestley, M. (1994). *Essays on Analytical Music Therapy.* Gilsum, NH: Barcelona.

Purvis, J., & Samet, S. (1976). *Music in developmental therapy.* Baltimore, MD: University Park Press.

"Rationale." (2016). In *Merriam-Webster online dictionary.* Retrieved from www.merriam-webster.com/dictionary/rationale

Reed, K. J. (2002). Music therapy treatment groups for mentally disordered offenders (MDO) in a state hospital setting. *Music Therapy Perspectives, 20*(2), 98–104. doi:10.1093/mtp/20.2.98

Reuer, B. (2005). *Music therapy toolbox: Medical settings: Strategies, applications, and sample forms for therapists.* San Diego, CA: MusicWorx of California.

Reuer, B. L., Crowe, B., & Bernstein, B. (1999). *Best practice in music therapy: Utilizing group percussion strategies for promoting volunteerism in well older adults* (2nd ed.). Silver Spring, MD: American Music Therapy Association.

Ridder, H. M., & Wheeler, B. L. (2015). Music therapy for older adults. In B. L. Wheeler (Ed.), *Music therapy handbook* (pp. 367–378). New York, NY: Guilford Press.

Rider, M. (1981). The assessment of cognitive functioning level through musical perception. *Journal of Music Therapy, 18*(3), 110–119. doi:10.1093/jmt/18.3.110

Rio, R. E., & Tenney, K. S. (2002). Music therapy for juvenile offenders in residential treatment. *Music Therapy Perspectives, 20*(2), 89–97. doi:10.1093/mtp/20.2.89

Ritholz, M. S., & Robbins, C. (1999). *Themes for therapy.* New York, NY: Carl Fischer.

Ritholz, M. S., & Robbins, C. (2002). *More themes for therapy.* New York, NY: Carl Fischer.

Ritter-Cantesanu, G. (2014). Music therapy and the IEP process. *Music Therapy Perspectives, 32*(2), 142–152. doi:10.1093/mtp/miu018

Robazza, C., Macaluso, C., & D'Urso, V. (1994). Emotional reactions to music by gender, age, and expertise. *Perceptual and Motor Skills, 79*(2), 939–944. doi:10.2466/pms.1994.79.2.939

Robb, S. (1996). Techniques in song writing: Restoring emotional and physical well being in adolescents who have been traumatically injured. *Music Therapy Perspectives, 14*(1), 30–37. doi:10.1093/mtp/14.1.30

Robbins, C., & Robbins, C. (1980). *Music for the hearing-impaired and other special populations.* St. Louis, MO: MMB Music. (available through Nordoff-Robbins Center, New York, NY)

Robbins, C., & Robbins, C. (1998). *Healing heritage: Paul Nordoff exploring the tonal language of music.* Gilsum, NH: Barcelona.

Roberts, M., & McFerran, K. (2013). A mixed methods analysis of songs written by bereaved preadolescents in individual music therapy. *Journal of Music Therapy, 50*(1), 25–52. doi:10.1093/jmt/50.1.25

Rogers, P. J. (2003). Working with Jenny: Stories of gender, power, and abuse. In S. Hadley (Ed.), *Psychodynamic music therapy: Case studies* (pp. 123–140). Gilsum, NH: Barcelona.

Rolvsjord, R. (2010). *Resource-Oriented Music Therapy in mental health care.* Gilsum, NH: Barcelona.

Ruud, E. (1980). *Music therapy and its relationship to current treatment theories.* St. Louis, MO: MMB Music.

Ruud, E. (1998). *Music therapy: Improvisation, communication, and culture.* Gilsum, NH: Barcelona.

Sabbatella, P. L., & Lazo, P. K. (2015, June). Child musical development and music therapy assessment: Designing an assessment procedure for children with developmental disorders. Poster session presented at the 2ⁿᵈ Nordoff-Robbins Plus Conference, London, UK. doi:10.13140/RG.2.1.3437.9605

Sadovnik, N. (2014). The birth of a therapeutic recording studio: Addressing the needs of the Hip-Hop generation on an adult inpatient psychiatric unit. In W. L. Magee (Ed.), *Music technology in therapeutic and health settings* (pp. 247–261). London, UK: Jessica Kingsley.

Sandrock, D., & James, M. R. (1989). Assessment instruments for music-assisted relaxation training. *Music Therapy Perspectives, 7*(1), 44–50. doi:10.1093/mtp/7.1.44

Scalenghe, R., & Murphy, K. M. (2000). Music therapy assessment in the managed care environment. *Music Therapy Perspectives, 18*(1), 23–30. doi:10.1093/mtp/18.1.23

Schaffer, H. R., & Emerson, P. F. (1964). The development of social attachments in infancy. *Monographs of the Society for Research in Child Development, 29*(3), 1–77. doi:10.2307/1165727

Scheiby, B. B. (1999). Music as symbolic expression: Analytical Music Therapy. In D. J. Wiener (Ed.), *Beyond talk therapy: Using movement and expressive techniques in clinical practice* (pp. 263–285). Washington, DC: American Psychological Association.

Scheiby, B. B. (2015). Analytical Music Therapy. In B. L. Wheeler (Ed.), *Music therapy handbook* (pp. 206–219). New York, NY: Guilford Press.

Schmidt, J. A. (1983). Songwriting as a therapeutic procedure. *Music Therapy Perspectives, 1*(2), 4–7. doi:10.1093/mtp/1.2.4

Schwartz, E. (2008). *Music, therapy, and early childhood: A developmental approach.* Gilsum, NH: Barcelona.

Shakow, D., & Rosenzweig, S. (1940). The use of the tautophone ("Verbal Summator") as an auditory apperceptive test for the study of personality. *Character and Personality, 8*, 216–226.

Shaw, J. (1993). *The joy of music in maturity.* St. Louis, MO: MMB Music.

Sheridan, S. M., & Kratochwill, T. R. (2007). *Conjoint behavioral consultation: Promoting family-school connections and interventions* (2ⁿᵈ ed.). New York, NY: Springer.

Shultis, C. (1995). *Music therapy assessment and initial treatment plan.* Unpublished manuscript.

Shultis, C. (1999). Music therapy inpatient psychiatric treatment in the 1990s. *Psychiatric Times, 16*(2). Retrieved from http://www.psychiatrictimes.com/articles/music-therapy-inpatient-psychiatric-care-1990s

Shultis, C., & Gallagher, L. (2015). Medical music therapy for adults. In B. L. Wheeler (Ed.), *Music therapy handbook* (pp. 441–453). New York, NY: Guilford Press.

Silber, F., & Hes, J. P. (1995). The use of songwriting with patients diagnosed with Alzheimer's disease. *Music Therapy Perspectives, 13*(1), 31–34. doi:10.1093/mtp/13.1.31

Silverman, M. (2012). Effects of group songwriting on motivation and readiness for treatment on patients in detoxification: A randomized wait-list effectiveness study. *Journal of Music Therapy, 49*(4), 414–429. doi:10.1093/jmt/49.4.414

Sinha, S., McDermott, F., Srinivas, G., & Houghton, P. W. (2011). Use of abbreviations by healthcare professionals: What is the way forward? *Postgraduate Medicine Journal, 87*(1029), 450–452. doi:10.1136/pgmj.2010.097394

Skille, O. (1997). Potential applications of vibroacoustic therapy. In T. Wigram & C. Dileo (Eds.), *Music vibration* (pp. 49–53). Cherry Hill, NJ: Jeffrey Books.

Skinner, B. F. (1976). *About behaviorism.* New York, NY: Vintage.

Snow, S. (2009). The development of a music therapy assessment tool: A pilot study. In S. Snow & M. D'Amico (Eds.), *Assessment in the creative arts therapies* (pp. 47–98). Springfield, IL: Charles C. Thomas.

Sperry, L., Carlson, J., & Kjor, D. (2003). *Becoming an effective therapist.* Boston, MA: Allyn & Bacon.

Standley, J. (2000). Music research in medical treatment. In *Effectiveness of music therapy procedures: Documentation of research and clinical practice* (3rd ed., pp. 1–64). Silver Spring, MD: American Music Therapy Association.

Standley, J., & Jones, J. (2007). *Music techniques in therapy, counseling, and special education* (3rd ed.). Silver Spring, MD: American Music Therapy Association.

Stegemöller, E. (2014). Exploring a neuroplasticity model of music therapy. *Journal of Music Therapy, 51*(3), 211–227. doi:10.1093/jmt/thu023

Steinberg, R., & Raith, L. (1985). Music psychopathology: II. Assessment of musical expression. *Psychopathology, 18*(5–6), 265–273. doi:10.1159/000284414

Stephenson, C., Long, J., Oswanski, L., Plancon, J. R., Pujol, K., Smith-Morse, T., & Gainsfera, M. (2008). *Music therapy clinical self-assessment guide.* Retrieved from www.musictherapy.org/assets/1/7/SelfAssessmentGuide.pdf

Stige, B. (2002). *Culture-Centered Music Therapy.* Gilsum, NH: Barcelona.

Stige, B., & Aarø, L. E. (2012). *Invitation to Community Music Therapy.* New York, NY: Routledge.

Stige, B., Ansdell, G., Elefant, C., & Pavlicevic, M. (2010). *Where music helps: Community Music Therapy in action and reflection.* Farnham, UK: Ashgate.

Summer, L. (1990). *Guided Imagery and Music in the institutional setting* (2nd ed.). St. Louis, MO: MMB Music.

Summer, L. (2001). Group supervision in first-time music therapy practicum. In M. Forinash (Ed.), *Music therapy supervision* (pp. 69–86). Gilsum, NH: Barcelona.

Tamplin, J., Baker, F. A., Macdonald, R. A. R., Roddy, C., & Rickard, N. S. (2016). A theoretical framework and therapeutic songwriting protocol to promote integration of self-concept in people with neurological disorders. *Nordic Journal of Music Therapy, 25*(2), 111–133. doi:10.1080/08098131.2015.1011208

Taylor, R. R. (2008). *The intentional relationship: Occupational therapy and the use of self.* Philadelphia, PA: F. A. Davis.

Thaut, M. (2000). *A scientific model of music in therapy and medicine.* San Antonio, TX: IMR Press, University of Texas.

Thompson, A. B., Arnold, J. C., & Murray, S. E. (1990). Music therapy assessment of the cerebrovascular accident patient. *Music Therapy Perspectives, 8*(1), 23–29. doi:10.1093/mtp/8.1.23

Treder-Wolff, J. (1990). Affecting attitudes: Music therapy in addictions treatment. *Music Therapy Perspectives, 8*(1), 67–71. doi:10.1093/mtp/8.1.67

Trevarthen, C., Aitken, K., Papoudi, D., & Robarts, J. (1998). *Children with autism* (2nd ed.; pp. 172–202). London, UK: Jessica Kingsley.

Turry, A., & Marcus, D. (2003). Using the Nordoff-Robbins approach to music therapy with adults diagnosed with autism. In D. Wiener & L. Oxford (Eds.), *Action therapy with families and groups* (pp. 197–228). Washington, DC: American Psychological Association.

Turry, A. E. (1997). The use of clinical improvisation to alleviate procedural distress in young children. In J. V. Loewy (Ed.), *Music therapy and pediatric pain* (pp. 89–96). Cherry Hill, NJ: Jeffrey Books.

Unkefer, R. F., & Thaut, M. H. (Eds.). (2002). *Music therapy in the treatment of adults with mental disorders* (2nd ed.). St. Louis, MO: MMB Music.

Van Bruggen-Rufi, M., & Vink, A. (2011). Home is where the heart is. In A. Meadows (Ed.), *Developments in music therapy practice: Case study perspectives* (pp. 569–581). Gilsum, NH: Barcelona.

Van den Daele, L. (1967). A music projective technique. *Journal of Projective Techniques and Personality Assessment, 31*(5), 47–57. doi:10.1080/0091651X.1967.10120416

Wade, D. T. (2009). Goal-setting in rehabilitation: An overview of what, why and how. *Clinical Rehabilitation, 23*(4), 291–295. doi:10.1177/0269215509103551

Wadsworth, B. J. (1989). *Piaget's theory of cognitive and affective development* (4th ed.). White Plains, NY: Longman.

Waldon, E. G. (2016). Clinical documentation in music therapy: Standards, guidelines, and laws. *Music Therapy Perspectives, 34*(1), 57–63. doi:10.1093/mtp/miv040

Wärja, M., & Klinken, H. S. (2015). KMR (Short Music Journeys) with women recovering from gynecological cancer. In D. Grocke & T. Moe (Eds.), *Guided Imagery and Music (GIM) and music imagery methods for individual and group therapy* (pp. 253–266). London, UK: Jessica Kingsley.

Watson, D. E., & Wilson, S. E. (2003). *Task analysis: An individual and population approach* (2nd ed.). Bethesda, MD: American Occupational Therapy Association.

Watson, T. (2002). Music therapy with adults with learning disabilities. In L. Bunt & S. Hoskyns (Eds.), *The handbook of music therapy* (pp. 86–114). London, UK: Jessica Kingsley.

Webster, J. (2016, May). Task analysis—The foundation for successfully teaching life skills. About.com. Retrieved from http://specialed.about.com/od/glossary/g/Task-Analysis-A-Well-Written-Task-Analysis-Leads-To-Success-In-Life-Skills.htm

Wheeler, B. (1981). The relationship between music therapy and theories of psychotherapy. *Music Therapy, 1*(1), 9–16. doi:10.1093/mt/1.1.9

Wheeler, B. L. (1983). A psychotherapeutic classification of music therapy practices: A continuum of procedures. *Music Therapy Perspectives, 1*(2), 8–12. doi:10.1093/mtp/1.2.8

Wheeler, B. L. (1987a). Levels of therapy: The classification of music therapy goals. *Music Therapy, 6*(2), 39–49. doi:10.1093/mt/6.2.39

Wheeler, B. L. (1987b). The use of paraverbal therapy in treating an abused child. *Arts in Psychotherapy, 14*(1), 69–76. doi:10.1016/0197-4556(87)90036-0

Wheeler, B. L. (1999). Experiencing pleasure in working with severely disabled children. *Journal of Music Therapy, 36*(1), 56–80. doi:10.1093/jmt/36.1.56

Wheeler, B. L. (2002). Experiences and concerns of students during music therapy practica. *Journal of Music Therapy, 39*(4), 274–304. doi:10.1093/jmt/39.4.274

Wheeler, B. L. (2013). Music therapy assessment. In R. F. Cruz & B. Feder, *Feder's the art and science of evaluation in the arts therapies* (2nd ed.; pp. 344–382). Springfield, IL: Charles C. Thomas.

Wheeler, B. L., & Williams, C. (2012). Students' thoughts and feelings about music therapy practicum supervision. *Nordic Journal of Music Therapy, 21*(2), 111–132. doi:10.1080/08098131.2011.577231

Whitehead-Pleaux, A., & Spall, L. (2014). Innovations in medical music therapy: The use of electronic music technologies in a pediatric burn hospital. In W. L. Magee (Ed.), *Music technology in therapeutic and health settings* (pp. 133–148). London, UK: Jessica Kingsley.

Wiger, D. E. (2012). *The psychotherapy documentation primer* (3rd ed.). Hoboken, NJ: John Wiley & Sons.

Wigram, T. (1997). The measurement of mood and physiological responses to vibroacoustic therapy in nonclinical subjects. In T. Wigram & C. Dileo (Eds.), *Music vibration* (pp. 87–97). Cherry Hill, NJ: Jeffrey Books.

Wigram, T. (2004). *Improvisation: Methods and techniques for music therapy clinicians, educators and students.* London, UK: Jessica Kingsley.

Wigram, T., & Dileo, C. (Eds.). (1997). *Music vibration.* Cherry Hill, NJ: Jeffrey Books.

Wilber, K. (1996). *A brief history of everything.* Boston, MA: Shambala.

Wilmer, H. A., & Husni, M. (1953). The use of sounds in a projective test. *Journal of Consulting Psychology, 17*(5), 377–383. doi:10.1037/h0055254

Wolberg, L. R. (1977). *The technique of psychotherapy* (3rd ed., Pt. 1). New York, NY: Grune & Stratton.

Wolfe, D. E. (1980). The effect of automated interrupted music on head posturing of cerebral palsied individuals. *Journal of Music Therapy, 17*(4), 184–206. doi:10.1093/jmt/17.4.184

Wolfe, D. E., & Waldon, E. G. (2009). *Music therapy and pediatric medicine: A guide to skill development and clinical intervention.* Silver Spring, MD: American Music Therapy Association.

Wood, M. M. (1975). *Developmental Therapy.* Baltimore, MD: University Park Press.

Wood, M. M., Quirk, C. A., & Swindle, F. L. (2007). *Teaching responsible behavior: Developmental therapy-developmental teaching for troubled children and adolescents* (4th ed.). Austin, TX: Pro-Ed.

Wooten, V. (2006). *The music lesson: A spiritual search for growth through music.* New York, NY: Berkley Books.

Wosch, T., & Wigram, T. (2007). *Microanalysis in music therapy: Methods, techniques and applications for clinicians, researchers, educators and students.* London, UK: Jessica Kingsley.

Wyatt, J. G. (2002). From the field: Clinical resources for music therapy with juvenile offenders. *Music Therapy Perspectives, 20*(2), 89–97. doi:10.1093/mtp/20.2.80

Yalom, I. D. (1985). *The theory and practice of group psychotherapy* (3rd ed.). New York, NY: Basic Books.

Zabin, A. H. (2005). Lessons learned from the dying: Stories from a music therapist. *Music Therapy Perspectives, 23*(1), 70–75. doi:10.1093/mtp/23.1.70

Index